FAB Diet
THE ALL NEW
Fat Attack Booster Diet

Rosemary Conley CBE is the UK's most successful diet and fitness expert. Her diet and fitness books, videos and DVDs have consistently topped the bestseller lists with combined sales of around nine million copies. Rosemary has also presented more than 400 cookery programmes on television and has hosted several of her own TV series on BBC and ITV, including *Slim to Win with Rosemary Conley*, which was first broadcast in ITV Central and Thames Valley regions in 2007, with a new series in 2008.

In 1999 Rosemary was made a Deputy Lieutenant of Leicestershire. In 2001 she was given the Freedom of the City of Leicester, and in 2004 she was awarded a CBE in the Queen's New Year Honours List for 'services to the fitness and diet industries'.

Together with her husband, Mike Rimmington, Rosemary runs five companies: Rosemary Conley Diet and Fitness Clubs, which operates an award-winning national network of almost 200 franchises running around 2,000 classes weekly; Quorn House Publishing Ltd, which publishes *Rosemary Conley Diet & Fitness* magazine; Quorn House Media Ltd, which runs rosemaryconley.tv, an online TV channel; Rosemary Conley Licences Ltd; and Rosemary Conley Enterprises.

Rosemary has a daughter, Dawn, from her first marriage. Rosemary, Mike and Dawn are all committed Christians.

D0273176

FAB Diet

THE ALL NEW
Fat Attack Booster Diet

Rosemary Conley

arrow books

Published in the United Kingdom by Arrow in 2013
10 9 8 7 6 5 4 3 2 1

Arrow Books
Random House UK Limited
20 Vauxhall Bridge Road, London SW1V 2SA

Addresses for companies within The Random House Group Ltd can
be found at www.randomhouse.co.uk/offices.htm

The Random House UK Limited Reg. No. 954009

A CIP catalogue record for this book is available from the British Library

ISBN 9780099580461

Cover photographs by Alan Olley
Exercise photographs by Alan Olley
Slimmers' 'after' photographs by Alan Olley
Food photography by Clive Doyle
Edited by Jan Bowmer
Designed by Roger Walker

The Random House Group Limited supports The Forest Stewardship
Council (FSC), the leading international forest certification
organisation. All our titles that are printed on Greenpeace approved
FSC certified paper carry the FSC logo. Our paper procurement
policy can be found at www.rbooks.co.uk/environment

Printed and bound in in Germany by GGP Media GmbH, Pößneck

Contents

Acknowledgements

I created my FAB Diet 12 months ago and if you joined Rosemary Conley Diet and Fitness Clubs during that time, you will have been following this diet. Because of the outstanding success of the diet in our classes I decided to write a book about it and include some of our members' testimonials and stories. I hope their experiences will inspire you. A massive thank you to the wonderful franchisees who run our classes for embracing the new diet so enthusiastically and motivating their members to achieve such success. A big thank you, too, to all our members for their emails, letters and cards. You have proved that the diet really, really works and you are all so inspirational! I still take my own classes on a Monday evening and in the 41 years I've been running classes, never have I seen weight losses like those achieved by my members who followed the FAB Diet and I've included some of their photographs in this book.

A very big thank you must go to Naomi Mayer-Baker for writing her blog. Naomi, who is a member of our online slimming club, described her weight-loss journey in her weekly blog. I was so enchanted by it that I asked her permission to include it in this book. I am sure you will inspire so many readers, Naomi. Thank you for letting me reproduce the story of your wonderful journey.

A big thank you also to chef Dean Simpole-Clarke for his delicious recipes, to Pauline Beanlands and Sue White for gathering together the testimonials from our members, to Anja Zeman for calculating the calories and fat content of the diet menus and recipes and to Diana Buchanan for all her support and help throughout the compilation of this book.

I am fortunate to work alongside one of the most inspiring fitness professionals and teacher trainers in the UK – Mary Morris. Thank you, Mary, for helping me put together the workouts for this book and for your continuing encouragement and expertise in respect of both the diet and the exercises. Thank you also to my wonderful daughter, Dawn, for her infinite wisdom in helping me create the diet. We work brilliantly as a team and Dawn keeps me on track when I'm working on a new diet.

As any author will acknowledge, the role of a book editor is golden. My wonderful editor, Jan Bowmer, is amazing and I want to thank you, Jan, for everything you have done to make this book so easy to follow and comprehensive. You are a joy to work with and you really are a star!

Thank you to Alan Olley for taking so much trouble to make me look my best in the photographs and also for making my successful slimmers look beautiful. Thank you to Clive Doyle for his food photography. I must also thank designer Roger Walker for making the book so easy to use and to Susan Sandon and Gillian Holmes at Random House for continuing to believe in me. Long may it continue!

Introduction

My Fat Attack Booster Diet was introduced to the members of Rosemary Conley Diet and Fitness Clubs in January 2012. We had the best January ever that year with a 30 per cent increase in new members compared to the previous year. Of course, part of the reason for this was that I was appearing on ITV1's *Dancing On Ice* in front of nine million viewers on a Sunday evening, but I think it was also because we had introduced a new diet that was incredibly effective while being so easy to follow.

I think my appearance on *Dancing On Ice* made folk realise it's never too late to get slim and fit and gave them the incentive to do it for themselves – I couldn't have succeeded in staying in the competition for six weeks if I'd been unfit and overweight. There's no doubt it's an incredibly physically demanding show and my years of teaching exercise certainly stood me in good stead. My body was also fairly flexible and my weight was at a healthy level. I was surprised how few aches I experienced and how much energy I found every day – but I was having the time of my life and had the loveliest skating partner in Mark Hanretty, who was a sheer delight to be with as well as being an amazingly talented coach and professional ice skater. I now have a passion for ice skating and for encouraging older folk to shed their excess weight and become fitter, because there's a heck of a lot of living still to be done after you turn 60!

It was due to the remarkable success stories we were seeing in our classes and in our online slimming club that I decided to write this book. Not everyone is able to join a

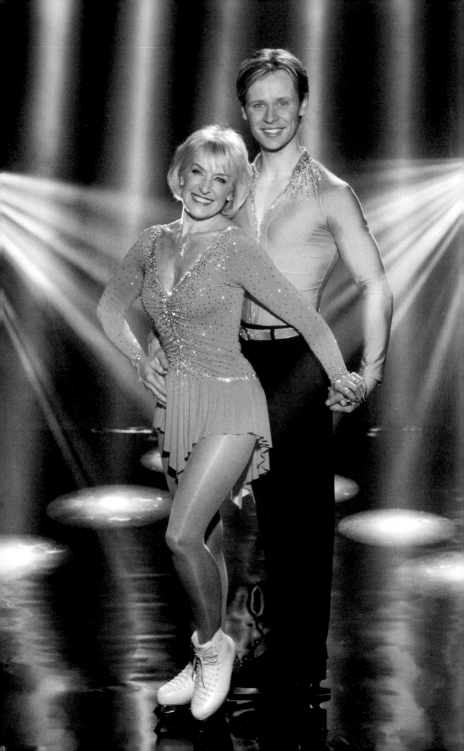

class or has access to a computer so I hope this book will show folk that weight loss doesn't need to be complicated. The great news is that you don't have to follow a very-low-calorie diet (VLCD) of around 600 calories a day or have meal replacements like milkshakes or powdery soups to see a fast weight drop. On my Fat Attack Booster Diet – or FAB Diet for short – you can eat healthy, low-fat, calorie-counted proper meals combined with some doable exercises that will fit into your daily life. Do this and you will slim down and tone up like never before.

I honestly believe this is the easiest diet to follow – ever! But don't take my word for it. Take a look at the 'before' and 'after' success stories included in this book and read the comments and letters I received from our members who all lost weight successfully and transformed their figures. These are real people who are living proof that this diet works. Our FAB dieters cannot believe the results they've achieved – safely, effectively and for life.

This diet works. Stick to it and you will be astonished at the results and you will feel amazing at the end of it. So, move it, lose it, love it!

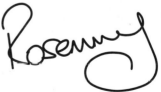

PS Throughout this book I've mentioned various products and services that we offer. All our products are very carefully selected and only included in my range if I honestly believe it will help whoever buys it.

Rosemary Conley and Mark Hanretty in *Dancing On Ice 2012* (ITV / Rex Features)

1
Lose weight fast and feel FAB!

Do you want to shed your excess weight fast and improve your health and fitness into the bargain? Well, now you can! In the 40 or so years I've been helping people to lose weight and get fitter I've never witnessed weight losses like those seen by our members after my FAB Diet was introduced to our Diet and Fitness Clubs in 2012. I've created diets before where trialists have lost a stone (6.4kg) in the first month but on my FAB Diet our members continued to lose weight at an amazing rate, with some managing a stone each month. The results were truly astonishing and yet the diet offers three meals a day of 'normal', everyday food. No powders or potions, and no gimmicks – just healthy food that YOU select from the many meal suggestions, together with some exercise that's within your capability, and you choose what you do. Put this magic combination together and you can achieve a slim and toned body, just like the slimmers featured in the photographs on pages 19–26. They all followed the diet and transformed their shape, size and health – fast! You can read their stories in Chapter 2.

This diet does what it says on the tin! It shows you how to boost your weight loss by attacking the unwanted fat on your body in a calorie-controlled, low-fat eating plan and effective exercise plan to help you achieve the figure and fitness level you've always dreamed of. And once you've lost your weight, I'll show you how to keep it off for good.

The beauty of my FAB Diet is that it's so versatile and caters for every taste and lifestyle. There are high-protein meal options if you like to follow a high-protein diet. Maybe you love your carbs? That's fine too, as I've included meals for those who love bread, pasta, rice and potatoes. Perhaps you have a sweet tooth? You'll find plenty of meal choices where a dessert has been included in the menu plan and, of course, there's a vegetarian alternative at every mealtime.

You can prepare your own meals, using the delicious recipes in this book, or for a speedier solution there are quick and easy alternatives for creating tasty meals using ready-made sauces – including my own Rosemary Conley range. And if you don't want the hassle of preparing a meal from scratch, you can select my Solo Slim® ready-meal options in the diet, which can be ordered through my website (www.rosemaryconley.com). All you have to do is pop a pouch of delicious 100% natural, healthy food into a microwave or empty the contents into a saucepan and heat on the hob. This really is the easiest diet ever.

And to make it really simple to select the type of meals you want, all the different meal categories are colour-coded so you can see your preferred options at a glance – for instance, all the high-protein options are in red, carbs are yellow, vegetarian green, and so on. See page 57 for the full key.

Your good health

Exercising regularly and eating a healthy diet that offers a balance of nutrients and plenty of fruit and vegetables will not only help you achieve a healthier and slimmer body and control your body weight, but will also help reduce your risk of developing serious conditions such as heart disease, high blood pressure, stroke, high cholesterol and type 2 diabetes. We all imagine these things won't happen to us but none of us is immune from disease and we should do everything in our power to reduce our risk.

In particular, the carbohydrate meal choices in my FAB Diet are ideal for diabetics as they are based on healthy low-Gi foods – that's foods such as oat-based or high-fibre cereals, wholegrain or multigrain bread, pitta bread, sweet potatoes and waxy new potatoes, basmati rice and pasta. Low-Gi foods help to lower the glycaemic index of a meal, which in turn helps to stabilise blood sugar levels. The beauty of low-Gi foods is that they also keep us feeling fuller for longer, thereby reducing hunger pangs – which is just what you want on a weight-reducing plan!

According to the charity Diabetes UK, eating a healthy diet can curb some of the complications associated with type 1 and type 2 diabetes. Untreated, diabetes can lead to blindness, heart disease, kidney failure and nerve damage. If you are a diabetic, losing weight will make a big difference to how your condition is managed. For people without diabetes, losing weight can also have a positive impact on their risk of developing the condition.

Diabetes UK advises that breaking down your daily food intake into three smaller meals, with snacks in between is useful for controlling the condition. So my FAB eating plan – which offers three main meals a day with a healthy mid-morning and mid-afternoon 'Power Snack' – is ideal for helping diabetics manage their condition as well as lose their excess weight.

Visit www.diabetes.org.uk for more information on diabetes, or you can watch Zoe Harrison from Diabetes UK

discuss diabetes on my free internet TV channel
(www.rosemaryconley.tv).

How does the FAB Diet work and why is it so effective?

No diet will work unless the total calories from the food and
drink you consume are less than the total calories you
spend in energy. If you eat less than you spend, you will
lose weight – it's a simple matter of physics.

Some foods have more 'fattening power' than others. As
fat has nearly twice the number of calories, gram for gram,
of carbohydrate or protein, cutting down on the fat in your
diet will be a huge help in your weight-loss progress. At the
same time, if you can spend a bit more energy by being
more active, you'll lose weight faster, providing you stick to
a calorie-controlled diet. But it's important to have enough
food to keep you feeling fuller for longer so you don't dive
into the biscuit barrel the first time you feel peckish! And
my FAB Diet allows you to do that.

I know that counting your daily calories is boring and
tedious. That's why all the meals in my FAB Diet are calorie-
counted, so you don't have to worry about that unless you
eat something outside of the recommended meals. I've
designed this FAB Diet so there's something for everyone,
and with plenty of variety in the menus offered you're
bound to find something to suit – whether you prefer cereal
or toast or fruit for breakfast or you like a sandwich or a
proper meal at lunchtime or perhaps eat only chicken or
fish for dinner. All the options are there for you to choose –
and repeat – to your liking.

To burn fat faster, as well as following the eating plan in
this book I ask you to do some aerobic exercise each day,
such as brisk walking, cycling or an aerobics class. Add in
some toning exercises three or four times a week and you'll

firm up and strengthen your muscles, which will give you a better shape. You can choose what exercise you do or you can follow the daily fitness challenges I've set for you in the first four weeks which will enable you to build up your fitness gradually. You may find it helpful to read Chapter 10 before you start the diet.

Three steps to successful weight loss

The FAB Diet is divided into three stages. The first stage is designed to kick-start your weight loss so you see quick results early on. Research has shown that if you lose a significant amount of weight in the early stages of a weight-loss plan, you are much more likely to continue. So, for the first two weeks, you follow the quite strict, 1200-calorie Kick-Start Booster Diet. You'll find the results of this initial effort incredibly encouraging. In trials, dieters lost an average of 7lb (3.2kg) in 14 days, so it's worth making the effort to stick to it.

In week three you move on to the 1400 Fortnight Diet, where your calorie allowance is increased to 1400 calories a day so you can enjoy an alcoholic drink and some extra treats. Then in week five you progress to Your Personal FAB Plan where your individual calorie allowance will be based on your basal metabolic rate (BMR), which is the number of calories your body needs to keep ticking over even if you stayed in bed all day and did nothing. This means that every bit of energy you spend moving around in your daily life and any other exercise you do will be fuelled by your body's fat stores and you'll burn more calories. (You can find your BMR by checking the charts at the back of the book.) Also in week five I've introduced a Fat Loss Booster day each week where on one day a week I ask you to be extra strict with your diet, sticking to

1200 calories a day, and to exercise more energetically, which will make a huge difference to your weight-loss progress.

Keep it off

Once you've achieved your desired body weight, it's vital to maintain it if you are to enjoy your new-found health, energy and confidence, and I will show you how to do this without feeling as if you are 'dieting'. Staying active and continuing to eat low-fat foods is the key to long-term success.

If you stick to the diet and exercise regularly, you will be truly amazed at your rate of progress and you'll look great and feel fit and fabulous. You are starting on a wonderful journey that will change your life.

2
Tried and tested

When my FAB Diet was introduced to our Diet and Fitness Club members in January 2012 I was staggered by the extraordinary results. Never before have I witnessed such fast and sustainable weight losses. Take a look at the photographs on pages 19–26. These slimmers all agreed to be photographed for this book in the hope they could inspire others on their weight-loss journey.

When Nicola Bishop joined my Diet and Fitness class on 12th March 2012, she wore size 20 exercise gear and weighed 13st 12lb (88kg). Her joints ached so much that she'd started using a walking stick and her doctor was about to put her on statins for her high blood pressure and high cholesterol. She felt self-conscious, tired and her self-esteem was at rock-bottom. Four months later Nicola had slimmed down to 9st 12lb (62.6kg), was wearing size 10 clothes and looked fabulous!

Nicola, 49, says: 'I couldn't believe how much I could eat on the diet and still lose weight. I stuck rigidly to the 1200-calorie Kick-Start Booster Diet for the first two weeks and was amazed to find I'd lost 13lb (5kg) in 14 days! I then followed the 1400 Fortnight Diet for the next two weeks and lost a total of 1st 8lb (9kg) in the first month.

'After the first four weeks I moved on to the Personal FAB Plan, where I was allowed more calories. I was worried that my weight loss would really slow down but I kept losing at a

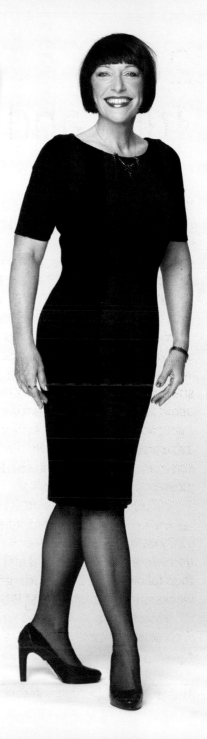

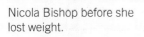

Nicola Bishop before she lost weight.

Right: Nicola after she lost 4st in 4 months.

SLIMFILE

Nicola Bishop

Age 49

Height 5ft 6in (1.68m)

Top weight 13st 12lb (88kg)

Now weighs 9st 12lb (62.6kg)

Total weight lost 4st (25.4kg) in 4 months

Dress size was 20 **now** 10

Bust was 44in (112cm) **now** 35in (89cm)

Waist was 43in (109cm) **now** 31½in (80cm)

Hips were 44in (112cm) **now** 36.5in (93cm)

Tops of arms were 13in (33cm) **now** 11in (28cm)

Above knees was 18½in (47cm) **now** 16in (41cm)

BMI was 31.3 **now** 22.3

rate of 2–3lb (0.91 and 1.4kg) a week. After four months I'd reached my goal of 9st 12lb (62.6kg). It was incredible!'

As well as sticking to the FAB Diet Nicola was determined to improve her fitness and started cycling the three miles to work. She added an extra couple of miles to her homeward journey in order to burn more calories! Today, after reaching her goal weight, she still comes to my weekly class and also power-walks for 15 minutes every lunchtime.

Nicola says: 'I'm more sociable now, my confidence is back and my fitness levels have gone sky high. I cycle 40 miles every Sunday and love it. I've been able to stop almost all my meds and my doctor is thrilled with my transformation. I feel 20 years younger, like a new woman. This diet, together with my exercise plan, has totally changed my life and I love the new me.'

Take a look at Nicola's 'before' and 'after' photographs to see the transformation.

Tracy Moore, 43, hated being overweight. When she joined my class on 16th January 2012 she weighed in at 17st 4lb (110kg). Her health was deteriorating, her joints were aching and she was getting chest pains – not good at any time in your life but particularly worrying for Tracy when she was trying to keep up with her energetic three-year-old daughter.

Tracy says: 'I felt I just couldn't interact with my little girl, and my weight made me feel so miserable, it affected how I felt about everything. I hated shopping for clothes and I always felt tired. I just felt so miserable.

SLIMFILE

Tracy Moore

Age 43

Height 5ft 11in (1.8m)

Top weight 17st 4lb (110kg)

Now weighs 13st 2½lb (83.7kg)

Total weight lost 4st 1½lb (26.1kg)

Total inch loss 54in (137cm)

Dress size was 22 **now** 14

Bust was 47in (119cm) **now** 40in (102cm)

Waist was 46in (117cm) **now** 36in (91cm)

Hips were 51in (130cm) **now** 43in (109cm)

Widest part was 52in (132cm) **now** 44in (112cm)

Left arm was 15in (37cm) **now** 12in (30cm)

Right arm was 16in (41cm) **now** 12in (30cm)

Left thigh was 30in (76cm) **now** 25in (64cm)

Right thigh was 31in (79cm) **now** 25in (64cm)

Left knee was 19in (48cm) **now** 17in (43cm)

Right knee was 18in (46cm) **now** 17in (43cm)

BMI was 33.7 **now** 25.7

Tracy shed 4st 1½lb in 6
months..

Inset: Tracy Moore before
she lost weight.

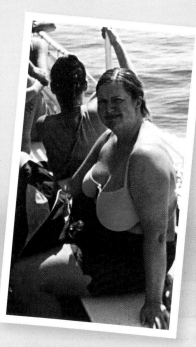

'I knew I had to do something as being overweight was taking over my life. In January 2012 I felt the time was right to take action. Rosemary was launching the FAB Diet in her classes and I was happy to give it a go. I couldn't believe how easy it was. I lost almost 2st (12.7kg) in the first two months and dropped three dress sizes. I was thrilled!'

By the end of July that year, Tracy – who is 5ft 11in (1.8m) tall – had slimmed down from a size 22 to a size 14 and now weighs 13st 2½lb (83.7kg). In six months Tracy lost 4st 1½lb (26.1kg) and 54in (137cm) from her body.

She says: 'The best thing is that my health has improved dramatically, I can run around after my little girl and we love going to the park together. I bought myself a size 14 leather jacket from French Connection and it felt so good – as if I'd won the Lottery! The FAB Diet is easy to follow and you eat "normal" foods, which makes it more of a way of life than a diet.'

Colleen Williams, 39, had reached a point in her life when she was so overweight she didn't want to face people. She says: 'When you meet someone you haven't seen in a long time you can see on their face how shocked they are at your weight gain. So you stay at home, miserable and bored, eating huge, man-sized meals.'

Colleen had been overweight since the birth of her son 15 years ago. Her weight had crept up to 17st 3lb (109.3kg) and her dress size had reached a size 22 before she decided to join her local Rosemary Conley class in Churchdown, Gloucester, in January 2012.

She also worried about her health. 'I was sure my weight was aggravating my asthma and migraines and was the cause of my sciatica. So I decided that 2012 was going to be different. My 40th birthday was looming and I made up my mind that I was not going to be fat in my 40s!

Colleen lost 6st 11lb in 10 months.

Inset: Colleen at 17st 3lb.

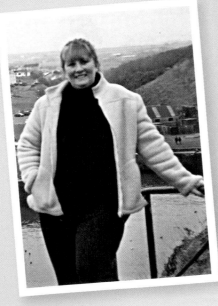

'I dreaded going out and about with my son and husband. Even when they were just walking, I found it hard to keep up with them. I'd have to stop, rest and take my inhaler and they'd have to wait for me.'

Within 10 months of joining the Rosemary Conley class, Colleen reached her goal weight of 10st 6lb (66.2kg). She now wears a dress size 10 or 12 and is fitter than she's been since her school days. She can walk up the steepest of hills with her husband and match him pace for pace. She hardly needs to use her inhaler for her asthma, her migraines are only an occasional occurrence and her sciatica has gone.

SLIMFILE

Colleen Williams

Age 39

Height 5ft 6in (1.68m)

Top weight 17st 3lb (109.3kg)

Now weighs 10st 6lb (66.2kg)

Total weight lost 6st 11lb (43.1kg)

Dress size was 22 **now** 10/12

Bust was 44½in (113cm) **now** 37in (94cm)

Waist was 41in (104cm) **now** 29in (74cm)

Hips were 40in (102cm) **now** 36½in (93cm)

Widest part was 44in (112cm) **now** 36½in (93cm)

Left arm was 16in (41cm) **now** 11½in (29cm)

Right arm was 16in (41cm) **now** 12in (30cm)

Left thigh was 25in (64cm) **now** 21in (53cm)

Right thigh was 25in (64cm) **now** 20½in (52cm)

Left knee was 20in (51cm) **now** 16in (41cm)

Right knee was 20in (51cm) **now** 15½in (39cm)

BMI was 38.9 **now** 23.5

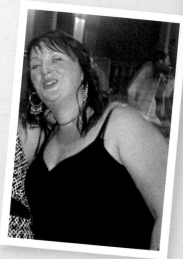

Inset: Naomi Baker before she joined our online slimming club.

Naomi as she looks today.

Best of all, she now loves going out socially with her husband and looks forward to deciding what to wear instead of dreading trying to find something to fit.

Naomi Baker, 39, gained weight after giving up work to have a family. During her last pregnancy with baby Leo she had gained more than 3st (19.1kg) and her weight had risen to 13st 4lb 4oz (84kg). Family commitments meant she couldn't get to a class, so she joined our online slimming club www.rosemaryconleyonline.com. She lost 2st 11lb 4oz (17kg) in 26 weeks on the FAB Diet and transformed her life, her figure and her health. Fascinated by the whole experience, she decided to write a weekly blog, which she sent to me to read. I was so enchanted by her weight-loss experience I asked her if I could include her blog in this book. You can read her personal story in Chapter 14.

What other dieters said

As well as the slimmers whose photos appear in this book there were many other success stories and I've included a selection of comments and extracts from letters I received from members of our classes.

■ Kirstie Davies, 24, from Suffolk weighed 15st 4½lb (97kg) when she joined her local class in January 2012. She wrote:

'The FAB Diet plan definitely works, even with my lifestyle. I would recommend it to any of my friends as it doesn't mean you have to put your life on hold – you can carry on the same as long as you just think about what you are eating and drinking.'

In just seven weeks Kirstie lost 1st 8½lb (10kg) and loads of inches – 5in (13cm) from her waist, 4in (10cm) from her bust, 4in (10cm) from her widest part and from her hips as well as 2in (5cm) off each thigh.

■ Zoe White, 21, joined our classes at the end of January 2012, weighing in at 15st 2lb (96kg). Zoe wrote:

'The diet is so easy to follow and I have really got into exercise. I am delighted that I've lost so much weight for my wedding.'

Zoe lost a staggering 1st 11½lb (11kg) in the first six weeks. By the end of June, she had lost almost 4st (25kg) in time for her wedding and her BMI had reduced from 35.4 to a much improved level of 26.4.

■ Jill Howard, 54, joined the Needham Market class in Suffolk at the end of January, weighing in at 14st 7½lb (92kg). She said:

'As crazy as it sounds, I am starting to feel like a human being again instead of a great tired old lump! My confidence has started to rise. I really enjoy the classes and everyone is so friendly, and they care – a great combination.'

In four weeks Jill lost 12lb (5.4kg) and shed 4in (10cm) off her waist and 2in (5cm) off her hips and bust.

■ Caroline Freil, from Northern Ireland, joined our classes in January 2012. She wrote:

'These are the changes I have made: cutting out the rubbish, watching my portion sizes, covering half my plate

with veg or salad, following the 5% fat rule, checking calories and labels before buying food, exercising more (walking and at class). If I have a bad day I write down the calories, which definitely helps me get back on track. Highlights so far: compliments from other people, have put away "fat" clothes as they are too big! I'm looking out clothes that have been in the back of the wardrobe for years, but which now fit. Love seeing the inches dropping off!'

In nine weeks Caroline lost 2st 1lb (13kg) and 18½in (47cm).

■ In just 12 weeks 18-year-old class member Liz King from Somerset lost almost 2st (12.7kg) and an amazing 7in (18cm) from her waist alone! Liz wrote:

'I can't believe how much weight I have lost. I'm happier and much fitter. I love it!'
Six months later, Liz had lost 4st 4lb (27kg) and her BMI has reduced from 35.9 to 25.6.

■ Class member Karen Blake, also from Somerset, joined her local class on 8th March 2012. Four weeks on Karen had lost 1st 5lb (8.6kg). She said:

'I never suffer from acid indigestion any more, I never have any knee pain and I feel so much happier and healthier!'

■ There's nothing like a forthcoming wedding to focus the mind on shedding a few pounds so when bride-to-be Hannah and bridesmaids Rachel and Nicky joined their local class in Cambridgeshire they brought enthusiasm, fun and laughter as they encouraged each other on their weight-loss paths at the classes.

As the date of the big day approached there was much excitement. Rachel wrote:

'I had my bridesmaid dress fitting on Saturday and it was massive (yay!). Just to think that I couldn't even get into it six months ago!'

Hannah and Rachel have each lost almost 1st 7lb (9.5kg), while Nicky has lost 2st 6lb (15kg).

■ Amy Berry, 26, from Suffolk also joined our classes to lose weight for her wedding. She wrote:

'I've tried pretty much every diet possible in the last eight years and have struggled with all of them and ended up slipping straight back into bad habits. I personally feel Rosemary's FAB Diet is amazing. It promotes good, healthy eating and exercise. The first few weigh-ins really inspired me to keep going and to stay on track. I lost 1st 5lb [8.6kg] in the first three weeks on the diet and in nine weeks I had lost 2st 6lb [15kg].'

■ Kim Hayes, 37, from Exeter started on the FAB Diet on 3rd January 2012, weighing in at 13st 7lb (86kg). By March she had lost 2st (12.7kg). She wrote:

'Having never followed any form of diet plan before I am surprised at how easy I have found it. I have really enjoyed cooking again and cook the meals in the FAB Diet for the whole family. I'm surprised at how quickly the weight is coming off. I am consistently losing 2–3lb [0.91–1.4kg] each week.'

By the time this book went to press, Kim had lost 3st 7lb (22kg) and was at her goal weight, slimming down from a size 18 to a super-slim size 10.

■ Also from Exeter is class member Sally Richards. Sally wrote:

'I think the FAB Diet is so easy to follow and very adaptable to different eating habits. I consider it a way of life now – not a diet – and it has made me a happy and healthier person.'

From January to July Sally lost an amazing 5st (32kg).

■ Nurse and shift worker Nicola Walters, from Bedford, works unsocial hours including long nights on duty. She started the FAB Diet and loved seeing the weight and inches dropping off. Nicola wrote:

'This is the easiest diet I have EVER done and it fits in with my difficult shifts brilliantly! The family love the recipes and they are SO delicious. You just can't go wrong. It's good all round!'

In six weeks Nicola lost 1st 4lb (8.2kg) and 29in (74cm) and has continued to lose weight at a very satisfactory rate despite suffering from a back injury, which means she has to take care when exercising.

■ Viv Debnam, from Sudbury in Suffolk, lost 2st ½lb (13kg) in eight weeks on the FAB Diet. She wrote:

'I feel ecstatic! It's so easy to follow, not like any other diet I've tried and, with the new healthier way of cooking, hubby has lost 8lb [3.6kg] too.'

■ Clare Strowger, 31, joined our classes in East Suffolk and lost 9lb (4.1kg) in her first week on the FAB Diet. In week two she was given her 'one stone weight loss certificate' at her class! Clare wrote:

'The diet is working for me as I love coming to class. I want to lose weight to make myself happy again and for my children – I don't want to be a fat mummy. We're also going on a family holiday so I would like to wear some nice summer clothes and feel great.

'The diet is perfect for me and has made me look at the calories and fat in all the food I eat, and also made me realise what rubbish I was eating before. I now understand how important portion control is too. Now that I'm eating little and often, I'm not eating all the naughty things I used to. I am doing lots more exercise. I love swimming as it makes me feel good and I really look forward to the exercises at the class as they are such fun – but also hard work!'

■ And in case you think the FAB Diet and our classes are only for girls, you couldn't be more wrong! Paul Anderson, 34, lives in Stowmarket. After following the FAB Diet for six weeks, Paul had lost 18lb (8.2kg). He wrote:

'I loved it from the start. I had tried a low-fat diet before so I knew I could lose weight, but the lower calorie allowance for the first two weeks was daunting – so I decided to see it as a game and I NEVER felt hungry. The exercise element was new for me – I have exercised before but never in any structured way and never in a group, both of which, I think, are vital to keep you on track and ensure the scheme works. More than any other weight-loss scheme, this

seems to be a logical mathematical process – it's not based on a wonder pill or special food, and it doesn't require a special mix of certain foods on one day or another – it's about "energy in" being less than "energy out".'

■ Another male member is student Jordan Galley, 17, who attends our classes in north Manchester. He wrote:

'At first I thought of Rosemary Conley classes as being for girls only and completely the opposite of what I wanted to do. But after the very first class I knew this was a brilliant choice for me. I have made many friends and am close to losing my third stone! I would recommend this diet and the classes to anyone.'

■ Ryan Lander, 18, who's a member of our Chadderton class in Manchester, lost 2st (12.7kg) in just seven weeks on the diet. He is currently away at university, but his class instructor told us:

'Ryan said he found the diet easy to follow. He is eating more fish and vegetables and taking more exercise. When he's at home he attends classes every Thursday with his sister, who herself has managed to lose 1st (6.4kg) in five weeks.
    'Ryan couldn't believe how easy it was to lose weight and how much better he feels and how much energy he has since he started eating healthily and doing regular exercise.'

■ Class member Hayley Kerry, 24, from Stowmarket joined her local class in January weighing 15st 4lb (97kg). In just nine weeks Hayley lost 2st 1½lb (13.4kg), of which 1st 3lb (7.7kg) was lost in the first three weeks! Hayley lost 4in (10cm) from her bust and her waist, 2in (5cm) off her hips,

2in (5cm) off each thigh and 2in (5cm) off her widest part. She wrote:

'I joined the Rosemary Conley class because I wanted to lose weight before my wedding in October 2012 and to be healthier. I've always been overweight – for as long as I can remember. Every year I seem to start a new diet but always give up after losing about a stone [6.4kg], because I get bored. I thought this diet would be better for me because of the exercise too. I think the FAB Diet has worked well for me because it allows me to eat little and often so I never feel hungry. The menu plans were a lifesaver. I didn't have to work out anything for the first few weeks – I just followed the menus. I used to eat way too much so Rosemary's Portion Pots® are very useful.'

■ Kerry Spurling joined our classes on 12th January 2012. She lost 3st 7lb (22.2kg) in six months and her BMI has dropped from 31.8 to 25. Kerry wrote:

'I can't praise the FAB Diet enough. It's the only diet I've managed to stick to – and I've tried a few! I also love the fact that it's not just a diet. You also get a workout thrown in at the classes. I really look forward to going even when I haven't been as good as I could have been. It's now a way of life.'

■ Twenty-two-year-old Amy Walker used to play a lot of sport but was forced to give it up after she got injured and had to have an operation on her knee. She ended up on steroids for 18 months and consequently gained a good deal of weight. She joined her local class in Wokingham in Surrey and started on the FAB Diet on 3rd January 2012, weighing in at 15st 10lb (99.8kg) and with a BMI of 40.2. In the first

12 weeks, Amy lost 2st (12.7kg) and by the time this book went to press Amy had managed to drop her weight by almost 5st (31.8kg) while her BMI is down to 27.8.

She said:

'The FAB Diet has been really good for me as I didn't know about portion sizes before and didn't realise how much I was putting on my plate. The diet also has taught me about the calories in food and the fat content. Following the diet has really helped me to lose weight as it gave me that first kick-start. It provides you with a variety of menu options and recipes. I found it very helpful to know which types of food were healthier choices. The diet worked for me as I stuck to the set calories for breakfast, lunch and dinner and I had the Power Snacks in the morning and afternoon, which meant that I didn't get as hungry for my main meals. I also used the exercise advice in the plan to help me increase my activity throughout the day. Seeing the weight come off each week has really motivated me to continue on the diet as I really want to reach my goal.'

Improved health

While I didn't set out to write a chapter on the health benefits enjoyed by followers of my FAB Diet, I feel it's worth including these very encouraging stories from some of our class members who have been following the diet.

High cholesterol

Geoff and Alison from Liverpool are a couple who slimmed down together. They joined our classes at the end of January. By the end of April Geoff had lost 4st 10½lb (30kg) and Alison had lost nearly 2st (13kg). Geoff suffers from asthma, high cholesterol and type 2 diabetes but after just three months on the FAB Diet he was able to come off his cholesterol medication. His diabetic nurse was amazed at the amount of weight he'd lost and was so delighted with his progress, she told Geoff that, with just a little more weight off, he could come off his diabetic medication too.

Heart problems

Sue Roberts, who attends our classes in Ryde on the Isle of Wight, lost 2st (12.7kg) on the FAB Diet. She wrote:

'Before I started at my local RC class I had limited mobility (arthritis in my hips, back and knees). I have been doing chair aerobics since the end of January and, although not perfect, I would say there is a huge improvement in my movement. I also have a slight heart problem and recently saw my cardiologist, who commended me on my 2st weight loss and asked how I had achieved it. When I told him I attended your classes, he was very interested and told me to keep it up as it was doing me the world of good!'

Blood pressure

Ali Miles, 47, joined our Waterlooville class in Hampshire weighing in at 10st 12lb (69kg). She lost 1st 8lb (10kg), slimming down to 9st 4lb (59kg). Ali wrote:

'I thought I would let you know my good news. I have been on two blood pressure tablets daily since 2008. I went for my six-monthly tablet review last week and due to Rosemary's FAB Diet, the weight I have lost and my new general fitness levels – as well as the fun we have at the classes – my doctor has stopped one of the daily tablets. He said that if my blood pressure stays stable in the next

eight weeks, he will stop the last one! He has also taken me off other medication I was taking for acid in my stomach, and told me to just take one when I need to, which has been only twice in the last six weeks. Incredible! The amazing thing is it doesn't feel like a diet or a chore. My doctor really does endorse the principles of Rosemary Conley, not just for me but he said it's an easy lifestyle choice and I have to agree.'

As this book went to press, Ali told us that her doctor has now taken her off her last blood pressure tablet.

Osteoarthritis

Pamela Tilney-Ellis, from Exeter in Devon, weighed 10st 12lb (68.9kg) when she joined one of our classes in January 2012 run by franchisee Fiona Dunn, who in 2011 won our Yummy Mummy Slimmer of the Year title. By the spring of that year, Pamela's weight was down to 9st 6lb (59.9kg), and the transformation in her health was remarkable:

This is what Pamela wrote:

'I am 77 and have had rheumatism since the age of six, following scarlet fever and several subsequent bouts of rheumatic fever. By the time I was an adult it had developed into osteoarthritis. Then, following a very stressful decade caring for my beloved husband who had vascular dementia, I developed an underactive thyroid. The result of this was rapid weight gain and despite balancing it with medication, the weight gain continued as my metabolism was not working correctly – there was little pineal gland function, meaning I did not sleep, plus an unreliable pituitary gland making everything out of sync!

When I heard that Rosemary Conley Diet and Fitness classes were starting up in Exeter I asked them if they could take me on – deformed feet and special shoes and all! They kindly and bravely agreed.

'Following the excellent and delicious Fat Attack Booster Diet, I immediately began to lose weight (though slowly because of my thyroid problem) but what I did not expect was the immense improvement in my mobility. I am now moving joints I have not moved for YEARS! At first I could only do a little, and those movements hurt and the crystals in the joints cracked! I am now managing to cope better. I can go up on my toes, which I haven't done for about 20 years. I can reach up better and I can step up a steep step. I can bend further and I can stand on one leg to dress myself. I also SLEEP MUCH BETTER and feel better than I've felt for years. As I started the classes at the beginning when they were first set up I've had the advantage of progressing with the routines as they were introduced, which has helped. I am VERY impressed with the way the instructors are trained – they really know what they are doing.

'PS: I can now get in and out of the bath unaided, which I have not done for 10 years!'

3
Planning for success

If you want to lose weight and get fitter and healthier, you must understand that you'll have to make some changes to the way you eat so you don't slip back into the eating habits that helped you gain weight in the first place. Switching to low-fat milk, choosing low-sugar drinks, filling half your plate with veg rather than too much protein or carbohydrates are all great habits to establish and ones that you can realistically keep up for life.

Most of all you will have to make some lifestyle changes. Obesity is not a curable disease but it is a manageable one. If you follow the diet and don't cheat – that means not eating treats or giving yourself excessive portion sizes – you will lose weight. Add into the mix some daily exercise that makes you slightly breathless and you'll speed up your weight loss. Diet and exercise are natural partners when it comes to controlling your weight and they can both make a real difference to your health. It's a winning combination.

Eat low fat
Although fat contains twice as many calories, gram for gram, as protein or carbs, it doesn't make the food you eat more filling or 'bigger', it just adds unnecessary calories.

When following this FAB Diet, select foods with only 5% or less fat – that's up to 5 grams of fat for every 100 grams of product. At the supermarket check the nutrition labels on the pack of each product before you buy. Look at the column that gives a 100g breakdown for the food, then check the figure for TOTAL fat content (see sample label opposite). All foods containing 5g or less fat per 100g can be eaten as part of this FAB Diet, providing you stay with your daily calorie allowance.

The fat content may be broken down into saturates and polyunsaturates, but for anyone on a weight-reducing diet this is not significant as it is the total fat content per 100g that is relevant in our calculations. If you follow the simple 5% fat rule, the fat content of your food will look after itself.

NUTRITIONAL INFORMATION

Typical values	Amount per 100g	Per 300g serving
Energy	443 kj/ 105 kcal	1329 kj/ 315 kcal
Protein	6.9g	20.7g
Carbohydrate (of which sugars)	11.2g (2.6g)	33.6g (7.8g)
FAT (of which saturates)	3.7g (1.7g)	11.1g (5.1g)

Even though there is a total of 11.1g fat in each serving, there is still only 3.7g fat per 100g (3.7%), making it a low-fat food.

As you can see, this food contains 315 calories per 300g serving. Keep this figure in mind when planning your menus.

Keeping an eye on the calories is just as important as checking the fat content. On the nutrition label look at the TOTAL calories (kcal) per serving, alongside the ENERGY breakdown, to keep tabs on your daily intake.

The 5% fat guideline is an extremely simple and effective rule of thumb, with no need to count or add up fat grams in each portion of food you eat. The only exceptions to this rule are lean cuts of meats such as beef, lamb and pork, which may be just over the 5% yardstick, oily fish such as salmon and mackerel, which may yield as much as 10% fat, and oats. These exceptions are made because these foods contain important nutrients.

Practise portion control

Eating too big a portion is one of the principal reasons why people fail to lose weight, even on the healthiest diet. It's easy to become complacent about your portion sizes and that's when the extra calories can creep in and slow down your weight-loss progress. General foods, such as pasta, rice, breakfast cereals, juice or alcohol, are the hardest to estimate by eye and research shows you can easily be seduced into serving more than you intend by using large plates, dishes or utensils. Combat this by weighing your food or using my Portion Pots® or some other measuring tool.

My Portion Pots® are handy tools for measuring everyday foods such as cereal, rice and pasta and make it incredibly simple to gauge your portion sizes accurately. The pots come in four different colours and sizes along with a quick guide as to how much each pot holds of a variety of everyday foods (for more information and to order go to www.rosemaryconley.com). However, in this FAB Diet I've done all the relevant calculations for you and also given the metric equivalent measures

Rosemary Conley's Portion Pots®

The quick and simple way
to measure your portions

blue 80ml

yellow 125ml

red 250ml

green 330ml

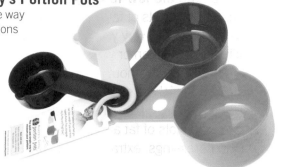

10 tips for low-fat cooking

1 *Go non-stick.* Use a good-quality non-stick pan or wok (with lid) and non-stick friendly utensils – wooden, silicone or rubber spoons and spatulas – to avoid damaging the surface.

2 *Preheat your pan.* Heat your pan to 'hot' before adding meat, poultry, fish or vegetables. Test by adding a small piece; if it sizzles, the pan is hot enough.

3 *Discard skin and visible fat.* Remove all visible fat and skin from chops, joints, chicken, etc. before cooking, and you'll save yourself hundreds of unwanted calories.

4 *Dry-fry.* When cooking mince, dry-fry it first and then drain it in a colander to remove the fat that has emerged. Wipe out the pan with kitchen paper to remove any fatty residue, then return the meat to the pan to continue cooking.

5 *Use vegetable stock for flavour.* When cooking rice, pasta and vegetables, add a vegetable stock cube to the cooking water. Although the stock cube contains a little fat, the amount that is absorbed by the food is

Prepare food the low-fat way

You can cut out lots of fat calories by making some simple adjustments to the way you prepare food. Invest in a good-quality non-stick pan or wok so you can dry-fry any meat, fish or vegetables without adding fat or oil to the pan. When making sandwiches, spread your bread with low-fat dressings in preference to butter or margarine and you'll save yourself lots of fat and calories. Branston pickle, low-fat salad dressings, extra-light mayonnaise, extra-light soft

---

negligible and the benefit in flavour is very noticeable and it does away with the need to add butter, salt or oil before serving.

6 *Replace oil.* Use soy sauce and balsamic vinegar or wine vinegar in stir-fries and salads in place of oil.

7 *Make mash low fat.* Mash potatoes with yogurt or semi-skimmed milk instead of butter, spread or cream.

8 *Spice up foods.* Garlic, chilli and other herbs and spices are great for adding flavour to dishes. Black pepper enhances any dish, so get a good pepper mill and buy your peppercorns whole.

9 *Use fat-free or low-fat yogurt.* Use 0%, 2% or 3% fat Greek yogurt instead of double cream or crème fraiche to flavour dishes, but never allow it to boil or it will curdle.

10 *Dry-roast.* Instead of roasting potatoes and parsnips in oil, parboil them with a vegetable stock cube for 5 minutes, then drain and transfer to a non-stick baking tray. Roast on the top shelf of a hot oven until golden brown (about 45 minutes for potatoes, 35 minutes for parsnips).

cheese, HP sauce, and horseradish sauce are great
alternatives that can be spread straight onto bread.

Plot your success

Making the decision to lose weight is a big step because it
involves thought and planning as well as willpower. If you
are to succeed, it's crucial to set yourself some goals. Goals
give us a focus. Sometimes our goals take longer to achieve
than we'd wish but that doesn't matter – so long as we get
there in the end.

Setting weight-loss goals requires some thought. Should
you set your desired end weight as your goal? Or should
your goal be to lose a stone at a time so that each 1-stone
loss becomes a goal in itself? Maybe your goal will be to get
from a size 18 to a 12? Or perhaps you have a more general
goal such as 'I want to lose weight this year'– which is an
admirable aim but not as motivating, as it won't be so easy
to determine when you've actually reached it.

Go for great goals

When it comes to weight loss, it's very easy to become
fixated on your ultimate goal but it's the journey that gives
the greatest thrill and I believe that small goals prove the
most rewarding. If you set too difficult a goal at the outset,
you will only end up demoralised if you fail to achieve it. A
shorter-term goal such as 'I want to lose a stone in the first
four weeks' is both achievable and realistic, but the most
exciting thing is that it won't take long.

Each small goal you achieve gives you the confidence to
set a new goal. Even if it takes you six weeks to achieve
your initial goal, it really doesn't matter – the most important
thing is to stay focused and to make a plan. But if you do
achieve that 1-stone loss in just four weeks, reward yourself

– maybe with a new pair of shoes, some luxury new make-up, a manicure, a special day out, or whatever other treat you fancy. Rewards are very motivating and the rewards that we enjoy on our weight-loss journey will help us to reach our ultimate goal.

Here are some goal ideas to get you thinking:

My goal is to...
- Lose a stone in ___ weeks
- Drop a dress size in ___ weeks
- Get into the next stone 'band' (say from 14 stone-something to 13 stone-something)
- Be able to walk up the stairs without having to pause halfway
- Manage to do the entire workout at my Rosemary Conley class rather than just the warm-up
- Be able to walk around the block in ___ minutes
- Get slim enough to wear my favourite _____ (skirt/top/trousers/jeans/dress)
- Do up my belt by a notch
- Be able to feel my work uniform fitting more loosely and comfortably rather than feeling it's 'stuck' to my body.

Timescale targets

It's always good to have short-term goals, long-term goals and ultimate goals. I am a real goal-setter and make lists of my aims and ambitions. I sometimes change or tweak those goals but they are nevertheless there in my mind.

Setting up our wonderful Diet and Fitness Clubs was a goal. Launching my *Diet & Fitness* magazine in 1996 was a goal. Building a TV studio was a goal. Being selected for ITV1's *Dancing On Ice* in 2012 was a goal.

Without goals we will flounder around, just existing, and that's a waste. If you want to be slim, healthy and fit, goals are essential. And rather than half-heartedly meandering with a mindset of 'Well, I would like to be a bit slimmer...' try to approach your weight-loss goals with the same focus and determination as an athlete.

Diet decisions

Once you've set your first goal, have a look at the menu plans in Chapter 5 and decide which meal options you prefer. Will you be preparing all your own meals or would you prefer to have my Solo Slim® ready-meal options – if it's the latter, all you will have to do then is buy some breakfast cereal and some fruit and veg to accompany your ready meals. Make a list of foods you plan to buy – and don't include those you should no longer be buying!

What about exercise? Will you follow the exercise plan in this book? When will you do it? What type of exercise do you fancy doing? What can you fit into your lifestyle? Turn to Chapter 10 to read about the benefits of exercise and how it will help speed up your weight loss. Then make a plan of the exercise you want to do, and stick to it.

10 golden rules for weight-loss success

1 *Take 'before' photographs.* Ask your partner or a friend to take photographs of you – from the front, back and side – before you start the diet. Then when you've lost your excess weight you can look back at these photos and realise how far you have come.
2 *Monitor your progress.* Weigh and measure yourself once a week and keep a record. This will provide the most encouraging proof of your progress.

3 *Eat three meals a day.* Make a decision to eat three main meals a day. You're much more likely to snack if you skip breakfast or don't eat a proper lunch.

4 *Plan ahead* so you know what you are going to eat for the week, or at least for each day.

5 *Shop wisely.* Make a list and stick to it. Don't be seduced by supermarket special offers. If you're buying other foods for the rest of the family, keep them out of sight once you're back home.

6 *Resist temptation.* Identify the foods you find difficult to resist and don't buy them! It's the only way to avoid temptation. If they're not in the house, you are less likely to eat them. Research shows that seeing food does prompt us to want to eat it even if we are not consciously aware of it. It's hard to avoid all the advertising for food products, vending machines and other food outlets when you're out and about, but don't make life more difficult for yourself at home.

7 *Get your five a day.* Eat plenty of fruit and vegetables as they are low in calories and fat, they help fill you up at mealtimes and keep you healthy. Make sure you have enough milk or yogurt to keep your bones strong.

8 *Go easy on alcohol.* After the first two weeks of the diet, if you want an alcoholic drink, go ahead and enjoy one – but in moderation only.

9 *Don't snack.* Apart from having a small 'Power Snack' between meals, avoid snacking altogether. Most snacks are high in fat so it's double damage when we eat them, and they're addictive. You only need to eat a biscuit with your morning coffee on one morning to be craving it again the next day. And who eats only one biscuit, anyway?

10 *Be active.* Don't underestimate the value of physical activity. The health benefits you'll enjoy from eating healthy low-fat foods in moderate quantities and increasing your activity will be enormous. You'll also have more energy, look younger, sleep better and snore less!

Love losing weight!

Learn to enjoy every day as you progress towards a new you! With every day that you eat more nourishing food and become more active, you are becoming a healthier, trimmer and fitter person. It is totally life-enhancing and life-changing. Even after the first week, you will see and feel a difference. Your clothes will become looser, you won't feel so tired, you'll sleep better, your mood will be lifted... and that's after just one week!

As soon as you start losing the weight, your joints won't ache so much, you won't get so out of breath, your heartburn will disappear and you'll find climbing the stairs much easier. Honestly, these benefits really can be enjoyed within a week or two of following a healthy weight-loss eating plan and increasing your activity levels.

Ways to stay motivated

- Think about your progress one week at a time. Measure yourself once a week to monitor your inch losses. Weigh yourself just once a week rather than daily for a more accurate gauge of your weight loss. Find an old skirt or pair of trousers that you were bursting out of at your heaviest and try them on every week. Appreciate how much looser they are every single week.
- Place the equivalent weight of what you lose each week in a bag, using packets of lentils or rice to represent the

weight you have lost. Lift the bag each week to realise how far you have come since day one.

- Write down in a diary at the end of each week all the positives you feel from losing weight. Keep reading them to remind yourself of the enormous benefits you are enjoying.
- Start to reprogramme your brain so it doesn't crave chocolate, cakes, biscuits, crisps, excess alcohol. Surely, they are worth trading in for the incredible benefits you will gain?

When you can see and feel the rewards for your efforts – your clothes will feel looser and you'll feel healthier – you know the diet is working and you are encouraged to continue.

Once you have got your head around all this preparation, you are all set for a new you. How exciting is that?

4
How to follow the FAB Diet

My FAB Diet is divided into three separate stages to maximise your weight-loss progress:

PART 1: Kick-Start Booster Diet
WEEKS 1 & 2

PART 2: 1400 Fortnight
WEEKS 3 & 4

PART 3: Your Personal FAB Plan
WEEK 5 ONWARDS

Weeks 1 and 2: Kick-Start Booster Diet

The first two weeks of the diet are quite strict to give your weight loss a terrific boost early on. You are allowed 1200 calories a day and I ask you not to drink alcohol just for this two-week period. Try to complete the daily fitness challenges I've included in the plan to help speed up your weight loss.

During these two weeks your body will respond very positively to the healthier foods you'll be eating and the extra activity you'll be doing, and the weight will drop fast.

Within a couple of weeks when you've maybe dropped a dress size or at least had to tighten your belt by a couple of notches, you'll realise how easy it is to lose inches, and

I'm confident you'll then feel totally motivated to progress to the next stage.

Weeks 3 and 4: 1400 Fortnight

After the first two weeks, your calorie allowance is increased to 1400 a day so you can enjoy an alcoholic drink and a treat or dessert each day. Your body will use up even more of your fat stores as you get used to eating more healthily and becoming more active. Your daily fitness challenges will become slightly longer and more challenging, to ensure you tone up as you slim down. By the end of the first four weeks, as long as you stick to the diet and exercise every day, I would expect you to have lost at least a stone (6.4kg), depending on how overweight you were in the first place.

Week 5 onwards: Your Personal FAB Plan

From week five onwards your daily calorie allowance is calculated according to your individual basal metabolic rate (BMR). This is the number of calories your body uses to keep your body ticking over – your blood circulating, body tissue renewing and repairing and your organs working – in any 24-hour period, without doing any physical activity. You'd burn this number of calories if you stayed in bed all day and did nothing. So, if you stick to a daily calorie intake that is equal to your RMR, every bit of energy you spend as you move around in your daily life, as well as any additional physical activity you undertake, will be fuelled by the calories deposited in your body's fat stores. When this happens, you cannot fail to lose weight – it's a scientific fact. The charts at the back of this book will give you an indication of how many calories you are allowed each day, based on your gender, age and current body weight.

As we get older our basal metabolic rate slows down, which is why we gain weight more easily – it's just that we need fewer calories for our bodies to tick over. If you are under 60, your daily allowance is likely to be more than 1200 calories a day, so you can still use all the menu options – just add additional foods to the basic meals if your calorie allowance permits (see pages 360–61).

Continue to boost your fitness and your calorie expenditure by exercising regularly. Now that you've completed all the daily fitness challenges in the first four weeks, why not take your fitness up a gear by following the Advanced FAB Fitness Challenge in Chapter 12.

After your terrific progress in the first four weeks, it's important to continue to maintain your weight-loss momentum at a steady and motivating pace. To help you achieve this, from week five I have introduced a Fat Loss Booster Day each week. On one day a week I ask you to consume only 1200 calories (as in the Kick-Start Booster Diet) with no alcohol or treats, and also to do 30 minutes of fairly energetic exercise on that day. Having one day a week when you are really strict with your diet and you exercise more vigorously will make a huge difference to your overall rate of weight loss.

Diet notes

Food prep
Cook and serve all foods without adding fat. Grill or dry-fry foods instead of frying in oil (or use a little spray oil) and cook vegetables, rice and pasta in water with a vegetable stock cube for added flavour.

Milk

You are allowed 450ml (¾ pint) skimmed or semi-skimmed milk a day for use on breakfast cereals and in teas and coffees. If you are allergic to or intolerant of cow's milk you may have soya or rice milk instead. If you don't drink much milk, you may substitute 125ml low-fat yogurt (max. 75 kcal) for 150ml (¼ pint) milk.

Bread

Choose low-Gi wholegrain, multigrain or stoneground brown bread. In this diet, one slice of wholegrain bread has 100 calories.

Breakfast cereals

Choose oat-based or high-fibre varieties, e.g. Sultana Bran, All-Bran, Fruit 'n Fibre, Bran Buds and Grapenuts, or ones containing natural grains such as Shredded Wheat, Special K and Weetabix.

Salad

Salad includes all salad leaves, cress, tomatoes and raw vegetables such as cucumber, peppers, carrots, onion, mushrooms, celery and courgettes, and may be served with any low-calorie, oil-free dressing, balsamic vinegar or reduced-salt soy sauce. Avoid pre-packed or ready-made salads with dressing as most are high in fat.

Fruit and vegetables

Aim to eat five portions of fruit and/or vegetables each day. One portion of fruit is one small orange, apple or pear or a regular kiwi fruit, nectarine or peach or 115g fruit such as berries or grapes (described as '1 piece fresh fruit'). In this FAB Diet, one portion of vegetables is approx. 115g. All vegetables should be cooked and served without added fat. 'Unlimited vegetables' means any vegetables except potatoes of any kind.

Gravy
Make gravy with gravy powder or low-fat granules.

Oily fish
For good heart health it's important to eat two portions a week of oily fish, e.g. mackerel, salmon, sardines, herrings, even though this exceeds the 5% fat ruling.

Drinks
Regular and fruit teas plus coffee made with water are unrestricted. Use milk from your daily allowance as required. All low-calorie drinks may be drunk freely. Water is also unrestricted.

Rosemary Conley cooking sauces and Solo Slim® soups and ready meals
All meals and soups in my Solo Slim® food range and my low-fat cooking sauces are made using 100% natural, fresh ingredients with no additives or E numbers. Thanks to their unique packaging method, they have a long shelf life and can be stored at room temperature with no need for refrigeration. They take only minutes to reheat – just pop the pouch in the microwave, or empty the contents into a saucepan and heat on the hob. See below for order details.

Rosemary Conley Solo Slim® Nutrition Bars
My Solo Slim® Nutrition Bars come in three flavours – Chocolate and Raisin, Ginger and Lemon, and Toffee and Apple. Each 30g bar is remarkably satisfying, particularly if

taken with a drink, and each has fewer than 100 calories and less than 5% fat. They make a tasty low-fat treat, and half a bar is ideal as one of your healthy mid-morning or mid-afternoon 'Power Snacks' that will keep you going until lunchtime or dinner. See below for order details.

Rosemary Conley 5% fat Mature Cheese

This is a really delicious low-fat cheese – it's the only low-fat hard cheese I have ever eaten that doesn't taste like low-fat cheese! You can use it in sandwiches or salads and it's also suitable for cooking. Available by mail order only (see below) or at a Rosemary Conley class.

How to order Rosemary Conley food products

All items in my low-fat food range can be ordered online at www.rosemaryconley.com or by phone on 0870 0507727 and are also available at Rosemary Conley classes.

5
The Kick-Start Booster Diet

Follow this diet for two weeks only, choosing from the low-fat meal suggestions on the following pages. All menus are colour-coded.

Each breakfast menu offers a carbohydrate-based meal **C** and a high-protein meal **P**, with vegetarian options **V**.

The lunch menu offers a carbohydrate option **C**, a high-protein meal option **P** and a Solo Slim® meal **S** as well as vegetarian options **V**.

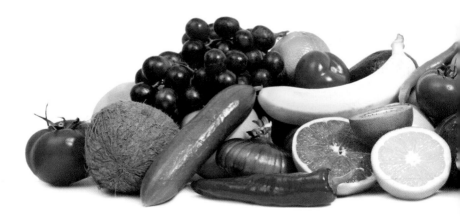

For dinner you have five options:

C = Carbohydrate-based meal

P = High-protein meal

V = Vegetarian meal (or vegetarian option available)

D = Dinner with a dessert

S = Solo Slim® meal

It doesn't matter which option you choose as long as the meal you select is something you fancy. All the breakfasts are 200 calories, all lunches 300 calories and all dinners 400 calories. The meals are interchangeable within each category so you can swap one breakfast for another breakfast or one lunch for another lunch, and so on. If you wish, you can repeat a meal on subsequent days, or you can choose any meal from the menus in Chapter 8, which offers many more meal suggestions. When making your choices, make sure you incorporate five portions a day of fruit and/or vegetables.

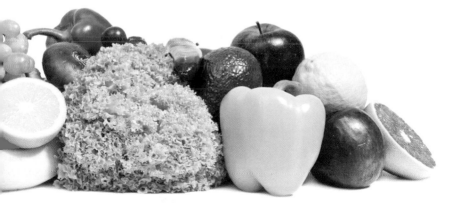

While you are following this or any other reduced-calorie diet, I recommend you take a multivitamin supplement each day just to be sure you are getting all the necessary micronutrients for good health.

Daily calorie allowance

Breakfast	200 kcal
Mid-morning Power Snack	50 kcal
Lunch	300 kcal
Mid-afternoon Power Snack	50 kcal
Dinner	400 kcal
450ml (¾ pint) skimmed or semi-skimmed milk	approx. 200 kcal
Total	**1200 kcal**

Weeks 1 and 2:
The Kick-Start Booster Diet

Diet notes

- During this two-week period, avoid alcohol and any extras.
- You can eat your main meal at lunchtime if you prefer.
- All meals are interchangeable within each category.
- If selecting a meal from another day or from the menus in Chapter 8, aim to incorporate five portions of fruit and/or vegetables per day.

Power Snacks

These are nutritious snacks designed to keep you going throughout the day, so I recommend you eat one mid-morning and one mid-afternoon, or at another time if you prefer. Do not exceed two in any one day.

Free calories

Regular and fruit teas plus coffee made with water are unrestricted – use milk from your daily allowance as required. All low-calorie drinks may be drunk freely. Water is also unrestricted.

Day 1

Breakfast

  1 green Portion Pot® (50g) Special K cereal served with milk from allowance and 1 tsp sugar. Plus 1 yellow Portion Pot® (125ml) unsweetened fruit juice

OR

 4 grilled turkey rashers plus 1 yellow Portion Pot® (115g) baked beans and 2 grilled tomatoes

Mid-morning Power Snack

 90g fresh blueberries

Lunch

 1 hard-boiled egg, sliced and made into a sandwich with 2 slices wholegrain bread spread with 1 dsp extra-light mayonnaise and filled with salad vegetables

OR

 2 hard-boiled eggs served with a large mixed salad tossed in oil-free dressing. Plus 1 kiwi fruit and 1 satsuma

OR

1 pouch Solo Slim® Low-Fat Carrot and Coriander Soup served with 1 small wholegrain roll (max. 150 kcal). Plus 100g fresh fruit salad

Mid-afternoon Power Snack

1 brown Ryvita spread with 20g extra-light soft cheese and topped with 2 cherry tomatoes

Dinner

 Mint Salsa Lamb Steak (see recipe page 201) served with either 1 blue Portion Pot® (50g uncooked weight) couscous or 200g new potatoes (boiled in skins), plus either a large salad tossed in oil-free dressing or 50g carrots and 50g broccoli

OR

 Braised Lamb Shanks (see recipe page 200) served with unlimited fresh vegetables (excluding potatoes)

OR

Roasted Vegetable Sausages (see recipe page 272) served with 1 × 200g baked sweet potato

OR

150g lean lamb steak, grilled, served with 200g vegetables (excluding potatoes) plus a little low fat gravy and mint sauce. Plus 1 Müllerlight banana and custard yogurt or other low-fat dessert (max. 100 kcal and 5% fat)

OR

1 pouch Solo Slim® Low-Fat Lamb Hotpot served with 200g fresh vegetables of your choice (excluding potatoes). Plus 1 piece fresh fruit

Daily fitness challenge
Take a 15-minute walk. Do 8 ab curls (with knees bent).

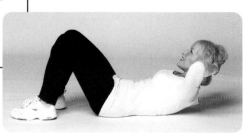

Day 2

Breakfast

 ⊘ Energy muesli (prepare the night before): Mix 15g (dry weight) porridge oats, 10g sultanas, 4 chopped almonds, 1 apple and 1 carrot (both coarsely grated) with 50g low-fat natural yogurt. Serve with additional milk from allowance if required

OR

Ⓟ ⊘ 2 eggs, scrambled, dry-fried or poached, plus 3 grilled tomatoes and 50g grilled mushrooms

Mid-morning Power Snack

Ⓥ ½ Solo Slim® Nutrition Bar or 1 small apple or pear

Lunch

 ⊘ 50g low-fat mature cheese (max. 5% fat), e.g. Rosemary Conley 5% fat Mature Cheese, served with 1 small multigrain bread roll (max. 150 kcal), halved, spread with pickle or extra- light mayonnaise and made into open sandwiches with salad leaves and sliced spring onions and cucumber

OR

Ⓟ 100g cooked chicken breast served with 1 small mixed salad tossed in oil-free dressing and 1 low-fat yogurt (max. 100 kcal and 5% fat)

OR

Ⓢ ⊘ 1 pouch Solo Slim® Low-Fat Mushroom Stroganoff plus either a large mixed salad or 2 pieces fresh fruit

Mid-afternoon Power Snack

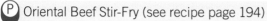 ½ Solo Slim® Nutrition Bar or 2 satsumas

Dinner

Ⓒ Ginger Beef Stir-Fry with Noodles (see recipe page 192) plus 1 dsp sweet chilli sauce

OR

Ⓟ Oriental Beef Stir-Fry (see recipe page 194)

OR

Ⓥ Sweet and sour vegetable stir-fry: Chop ½ onion, ½ red pepper and 1 celery stick and dry-fry with 50g sliced mushrooms, handful of mangetout and baby corn until soft. Add 125g (1 portion) low-fat sweet and sour sauce. Serve with 1 blue Portion Pot® (55g dry weight) boiled basmati rice and a little soy sauce

OR

Ⓓ Any low-fat stir-fry ready meal, e.g. beef stir-fry or similar (max. 350 kcal and 5% fat) served with 150g beansprouts or mangetout. Plus 1 Hartley's Low Sugar Jelly (max. 10 kcal) and 120g fresh fruit salad, or other low-fat dessert of your choice (max. 70 kcal and 5% fat)

OR

Ⓢ 1 pouch Solo Slim® Low-Fat Beef Meatballs and Potato served 100g carrots and 100g broccoli or cabbage. Plus 2 satsumas or kiwi fruits

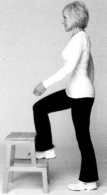

> **Daily fitness challenge**
> Walk briskly for 15 minutes. Walk up and down stairs twice consecutively.

Day 3

Breakfast

 1 slice toasted wholegrain bread spread with 2 tsp marmalade, jam or honey. Plus ½ grapefruit sprinkled with granulated sweetener

OR

 200g 2% fat Greek yogurt served with 100g fresh blueberries or raspberries

Mid-morning Power Snack

 12 seedless grapes

Lunch

100g tinned tuna (in brine or spring water), drained, served with 1 wholemeal pitta bread plus salad and 1 dsp low-fat salad dressing

OR

100g tinned tuna (in brine or spring water), drained, served with small mixed salad tossed in oil-free dressing. Plus 1 blue Portion Pot® (80g) low-fat fruit yogurt and 1 red Portion Pot® (115g) raspberries

OR

 1 pouch Solo Slim® Low-Fat Chunky Vegetable Soup served with 1 small wholegrain bread roll (max. 150 kcal). Plus 1 satsuma or kiwi fruit

Mid-afternoon Power Snack

12 cherry tomatoes

Dinner

2 low-fat beef or pork sausages (max. 5% fat), grilled, served with 1 red Portion Pot® (250g) mashed sweet potato plus 100g spring greens or sliced cabbage, 100g cauliflower or broccoli and a little low-fat gravy

OR

2 low-fat beef or pork sausages, grilled, served with 1 yellow Portion Pot® (115g) baked beans, 200g tinned tomatoes boiled until reduced plus unlimited grilled or boiled mushrooms

OR

2 Quorn sausages served with 1 red Portion Pot® (250g) mashed sweet potato, plus 100g spring greens or sliced cabbage, 100g cauliflower or broccoli and a little low-fat gravy

OR

2 low-fat sausages, grilled, served with 1 yellow Portion Pot® (100g) mashed sweet potato, plus 100g each spring greens or cabbage, 100g cauliflower or broccoli and a little low-fat gravy. Plus 1 low-sugar jelly, e.g. Hartley's (max. 10 kcal) served with 1 × 100ml scoop low-fat (max. 5% fat) ice cream (e.g. Wall's Soft Scoop) or other low-fat pudding (max. 75 kcal and 5% fat)

OR

1 pouch Solo Slim® Low-Fat Sausage Casserole served with 100g each cabbage and cauliflower

---

Daily fitness challenge
Do 20 minutes of aerobic exercise (brisk walk, class or DVD).

Day 4

Breakfast

 Soak 15g All-Bran overnight in 100g low-fat natural yogurt with 4 chopped almonds, 10 sultanas and 1 tsp honey. Serve with a little milk from allowance if required

OR

 1 egg, boiled or poached, served with 75g wafer-thin ham or Quorn Deli Ham Style Slices and 1 tomato, sliced. Plus ½ fresh grapefruit sprinkled with granulated sweetener if required

Mid-morning Power Snack

 200g fresh melon

Lunch

 1 yellow Portion Pot® (115g) baked beans served with 1 × 200g potato baked in its skin plus a large salad tossed in oil-free dressing

OR

 1 yellow Portion Pot® (115g) baked beans served with 2 well-grilled rashers lean bacon and 50g grilled mushrooms

OR

1 pouch Solo Slim® Low-Fat Spicy Mixed Bean Soup plus 2 Ryvitas spread with extra-light soft cheese and topped with sliced cucumber and tomato

Mid-afternoon Power Snack

15g raisins or sultanas

Dinner

 100g salmon steak, grilled, steamed or microwaved, served with 100g new potatoes (boiled in skins) plus 100g mangetout and 1 tsp Thai sweet chilli dipping sauce mixed with 1 dsp extra-light mayonnaise

OR

 Chinese Salmon Steaks with Stir-Fried Vegetables (see recipe page 235)

OR

 1 low-fat pizza (max. 350 kcal and 5% fat) served with a mixed salad tossed in oil-free dressing

OR

80g salmon steak, grilled, steamed or microwaved, served with 100g mangetout and 1 tsp Thai sweet chilli dipping sauce mixed with 1 dsp extra-light mayonnaise. Plus Eton Mess: 1 meringue basket, broken up, mixed with 1 tbsp 2% fat Greek yogurt and 10 fresh raspberries, or other low-fat dessert (max. 70 kcal and 5% fat)

OR

1 pouch Solo Slim® Low-Fat Leek and Potato Soup plus 1 pouch Solo Slim® Low-Fat Moroccan Spiced Chickpea Tagine

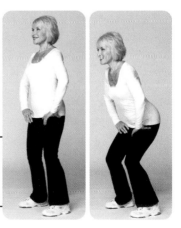

Daily fitness challenge
Walk briskly for 20 minutes.
Do 2 sets of 8 squats.

Day 5

Breakfast

 1 egg, boiled or poached, served on 1 slice toasted wholegrain bread spread with Marmite. Plus 200g melon

OR

200g 2% fat Greek yogurt served with 100g fresh strawberries

Mid-morning Power Snack

100g fresh pineapple

Lunch

115g cooked shelled prawns served with 1 low-fat tortilla wrap (max. 130 kcal and 5% fat) spread with 2 tsp Thai sweet chilli dipping sauce and filled with chopped peppers, cherry tomatoes, rocket leaves, spring onions

OR

 115g cooked shelled prawns served with large mixed salad tossed in 2 dsp low-fat thousand island dressing. Plus 1 low-fat yogurt (max. 80 kcal and 5% fat)

OR

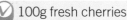 1 pouch Solo Slim® Vegetable Curry. Plus 1 Solo Slim® Nutrition Bar and 1 satsuma or kiwi fruit

Mid-afternoon Power Snack

100g fresh cherries

Dinner

 Chicken Korma (see recipe page 214) served with 1 blue Portion Pot® (55g dry weight) boiled basmati rice

OR

 Chicken Korma (as above recipe) served with a side salad, no rice. Plus 50g low-fat mature cheese (max. 5% fat), chopped and served with 1 small apple, sliced, 3 sticks celery, chopped, and 5 seedless grapes

OR

 Chicken Korma (as above recipe, but use Quorn Chicken Style fillets, or similar, instead of regular chicken). Serve with 1 blue Portion Pot® (55g dry weight) boiled basmati rice

OR

 Chicken Korma (as above recipe) served with 30g (dry weight) boiled basmati rice. Plus 1 low fat dessert (max. 100 kcal and 5% fat)

OR

 1 pouch Solo Slim® Low-Fat Chicken Korma plus 100g beansprouts and 1 mini pitta bread

Daily fitness challenge
Walk briskly for 25 minutes.
Do 2 sets of 8 ab
curls (with knees
bent).

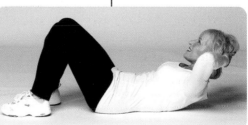

Day 6

Breakfast

 1 red Portion Pot® (50g) any bran cereal (e.g. Sultana Bran, All-Bran, bran flakes) served with milk from allowance and 1 tsp sugar or 1 sliced small apple

OR

75g smoked salmon plus 1 scrambled egg made using milk from allowance

Mid-morning Power Snack

1 fun-sized mini banana

Lunch

 100g cooked chicken breast (no skin) or Quorn Deli Chicken Deli Style Slices, served with 200g stir-fry vegetables, dry-fried with a little soy sauce. Plus 150g fresh fruit

OR

 100g cooked chicken breast (no skin) or Quorn Deli Chicken Style Slices served with large mixed salad plus 2 dsp low-fat Caesar dressing and topped with 20g shaved low-fat mature cheese (max. 5% fat)

OR

1 pouch Solo Slim® Low-Fat Chicken and Mushroom Risotto. Plus 1 satsuma or plum

Mid-afternoon Power Snack

100g fresh cherries

Dinner

(C) Pork and Leek Casserole (see recipe page 207) served with 1 yellow Portion Pot® (100g) mashed sweet potato and unlimited green vegetables

OR

(P) Melon and Parma ham cocktail: 200g sliced melon mixed with 28g Parma ham. Plus Pork and Leek Casserole (as above recipe) served with 200g fresh vegetables of your choice (excluding potatoes)

OR

(V) 1 green Portion Pot® (52g dry weight) spaghetti, boiled with a vegetable stock cube, served with ½ pot (175g) fresh tomato-based pasta sauce (max. 5% fat) and topped with 20g grated low-fat mature cheese (max. 5% fat). Plus 1 low-fat yogurt or fromage frais (max. 100 kcal and 5% fat)

OR

(D) 125g roast pork served with 200g vegetables of your choice (excluding potatoes) and a little gravy made without fat. Plus 1 × 25g slice fat-free Swiss roll served with 50g low-fat custard, or any other low-fat pudding (max. 130 kcal and 5% fat)

OR

(S) 1 pouch Solo Slim® Low-Fat Leek and Potato Soup, plus 1 pouch Solo Slim® Low-Fat Pork Meatballs with Smokey Beans. Plus 1 kiwi fruit or satsuma

---

Daily fitness challenge
Do 30 minutes of energetic chores such as car washing, housework or gardening.

Day 7

Breakfast

 1 slice toasted wholegrain bread topped with 200g tinned tomatoes boiled until reduced, plus 2 grilled turkey rashers or Quorn Bacon Style Rashers

OR

2 grilled turkey rashers served with 1 dry-fried or scrambled egg, 100g sliced mushrooms, grilled or dry-fried, and 200g tinned tomatoes boiled until reduced

Mid-morning Power Snack

 Vegetable nibble box: 80g carrot, 60g cucumber and 2 sticks celery cut into crudités plus 2 cherry tomatoes

Lunch

Pasta salad: 1 yellow Portion Pot® (45g uncooked weight) pasta shapes, cooked and cooled, then mixed with 100g tinned tuna (in brine or spring water), drained, or 100g Chicken Deli Slices, chopped, plus shredded lettuce, chopped cucumber, tomatoes and spring onions mixed with oil-free salad dressing

OR

200g tinned tuna (in brine or spring water), drained, served with shredded lettuce, chopped cucumber, tomatoes and spring onions mixed with oil-free salad dressing

OR

 1 pouch Solo Slim® Low-Fat Lentil Soup served with 1 wholemeal pitta bread. Plus 100g fresh fruit salad

Mid-afternoon Power Snack

50g blueberries topped with 1 dsp low-fat yogurt

Dinner

Turkey Spaghetti (see recipe page 228) served with a large mixed salad and 2 dsp low-fat dressing

OR

Turkey stir-fry with ginger: Chop 100g turkey breast (no skin) into bite-sized pieces and dry-fry in a non-stick pan with ½ crushed garlic clove. When the turkey has changed colour and is almost cooked through, add 1 chopped red or green pepper, 1 chopped celery stick, ½ chopped red onion, 25g mushrooms and 50g mangetout and dry-fry quickly but do not overcook. Just before serving add 1 tsp grated fresh ginger, soy sauce to taste and 1 tsp fresh coriander and heat through

OR

 Garlic Mushroom Spelt Spaghetti (see recipe page 259) served with a large salad. Plus 100g fresh fruit salad

OR

Turkey Spaghetti (see recipe page 228). Plus 100ml Ben & Jerry's frozen yogurt (any flavour) or any other low-fat dessert (max. 150 kcal and 5% fat)

OR

 1 pouch Solo Slim® Low-Fat Butternut Squash Soup, plus 1 pouch Solo Slim® Low-Fat Tomato and Vegetable Pasta served with a large side salad

---

Daily fitness challenge
Do 30 minutes of aerobic exercise (class or DVD) or play an outdoor game such as football or tennis for 30–40 minutes.

Day 8

Breakfast

 2 bananas

OR

 3 low-fat pork, beef or Quorn sausages, grilled, served with 2 grilled halved tomatoes

Mid-morning Power Snack

 1 rice cake spread with 20g extra-light soft cheese and 2 slices cucumber

Lunch

100g cooked pastrami served with 1 slice wholegrain bread spread with extra-light mayonnaise and made into an open sandwich with pickled gherkins and additional salad

OR

100g cooked pastrami served with large mixed salad tossed in oil-free dressing plus 50g mixed pickles. Plus 1 low-fat yogurt (max. 100 kcal and 5% fat)

OR

 1 pouch Solo Slim® Low-Fat Pea and Mint Soup served with 1 small wholegrain bread roll (max. 150 kcal)

Mid-afternoon Power Snack

3 dried apricots

Dinner

 Chilli Con Carne (see recipe page 196) served with 1 yellow Portion Pot® (cooked weight) boiled basmati rice

OR

 Chilli Con Carne (as above recipe) served with salad tossed in oil-free dressing, no rice. Plus 1 low-fat yogurt (max. 100 kcal and 5% fat)

OR

 Vegetarian chilli (ready meal or tinned version) served with 1 blue Portion Pot® (55g dry weight) boiled basmati rice plus a small salad

OR

 Chilli Con Carne (as above recipe) served with salad tossed in oil-free dressing, no rice. Plus 1 × 123g pot Dole Fruit Jelly or other low-fat dessert (max. 100 kcal and 5% fat)

OR

 1 pouch Solo Slim® Low-Fat Chilli and Rice. Plus 1 Ambrosia Jelly Pud (jelly with custard) or other low-fat dessert (max. 130 kcal and 5% fat)

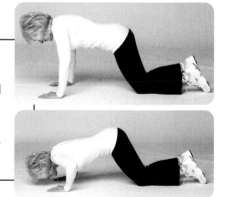

Daily fitness challenge
Walk up and down stairs 4 times consecutively and then do it again later in the day.
Do 2 sets of 6 semi press-ups (with knees bent).

Day 9

Breakfast

 1 blue Portion Pot® (35g dry weight) porridge oats, cooked in water and served with milk from allowance plus 1 tsp runny honey and 1 kiwi fruit

OR

2-egg omelette (made using milk from allowance) dry-fried and filled with 50g sliced mushrooms and 20g wafer-thin ham or Quorn Deli Ham Style Slices

Mid-morning Power Snack

20g wafer-thin ham or Quorn Deli Ham Style Slices plus 1 sliced tomato, 2 slices cucumber and a few salad leaves

Lunch

 100g tikka-flavoured cooked chicken breast chopped and mixed with 50g (cooked weight) boiled basmati rice, unlimited chopped salad vegetables and 20g sultanas. Add 2 dsp extra-light mayonnaise mixed with 1 tsp mild curry powder and chopped coriander

OR

120g cooked chicken breast (no skin) or Quorn Deli Chicken Slices served with a Waldorf salad: Mix 1 chopped apple, 2 chopped celery sticks, 15g sultanas, 4 chopped walnut halves and shredded lettuce leaves with 1 dsp extra-light mayonnaise and 1 dsp low-fat natural yogurt

OR

1 pouch Solo Slim® Low-Fat Tomato and Chilli Risotto served with a large mixed salad tossed in oil-free dressing

Mid-afternoon Power Snack

 ½ fresh mango (approx. 80g)

Dinner

 200g white fish steamed, grilled or baked, served with 1 yellow Portion Pot® (100g) mashed sweet potato and unlimited green vegetables plus ¼ pack Colman's Parsley Sauce mix made up with milk (in addition to allowance)

OR

Ⓟ 250g white fish steamed, grilled or baked, served with 300g vegetables of your choice (excluding potatoes) plus ¼ pack Colman's Parsley Sauce mix made up with milk (in addition to allowance)

OR

Ⓥ Crushed Bean Rigatoni (see recipe page 254) served with a large salad. Plus 1 piece fresh fruit

OR

 100g white fish, steamed, grilled or baked, served with 115g new potatoes (boiled in skins), 200g additional green vegetables, plus ¼ pack Colman's Parsley Sauce mix (made up with milk from allowance). Plus 1 scoop Wall's Soft Scoop Light Ice Cream topped with 100g sliced strawberries

OR

③ 1 pouch Solo Slim® Low-Fat Beef Bolognese plus a large mixed salad tossed in oil-free dressing. Plus 1 piece fresh fruit

Daily fitness challenge
Take 2 × 15-minute brisk walks during the day. Do 2 sets of 8 side leg raises on each leg.

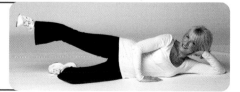

Day 10

Breakfast

 1 crumpet, toasted, topped with 2 dsp 2% fat Greek yogurt, 1 tsp strawberry or raspberry jam and 100g sliced strawberries

OR

1 2-egg omelette (using milk from allowance), dry-fried and filled with 25g low-fat mature cheese (max. 5% fat) and 4 cherry tomatoes

Mid-morning Power Snack

 200g fresh raspberries

Lunch

1 low-fat tortilla wrap spread with 1 dsp Thai sweet chilli dipping sauce and filled with either 50g tuna or prawns plus chopped salad (e.g. peppers, celery, spring onions, cherry tomatoes, cucumber) and shredded rocket leaves

OR

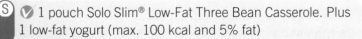 150g tinned tuna or cooked shelled prawns served with a large mixed salad tossed in oil-free dressing plus 1 dsp extra-light mayonnaise or Thai sweet chilli dipping sauce

OR

 1 pouch Solo Slim® Low-Fat Three Bean Casserole. Plus 1 low-fat yogurt (max. 100 kcal and 5% fat)

Mid-afternoon Power Snack

1 large orange

Dinner

 120g rump steak, grilled, served with 100g low-fat oven chips (max. 5% fat) plus 2 tomatoes, halved and grilled, 50g grilled mushrooms and a small green salad

OR

 175g rump steak, grilled, served with 1 blue Portion Pot® (75g) tomato salsa plus a large mixed salad and 1 tomato, halved and grilled

OR

 1 Quorn Peppered Steak served with 100g low-fat oven chips (max. 5% fat) plus 2 grilled sliced tomatoes, 50g grilled mushrooms and a large mixed salad tossed in oil-free dressing. Plus 100g fresh fruit salad

OR

Ⓓ 120g rump steak, grilled, served with a large mixed salad tossed in oil-free dressing plus 2 tomatoes, halved and grilled. Plus 1 meringue basket topped with 1 blue Portion Pot® 80g 0% fat Greek yogurt and 1 yellow Portion Pot® (70g) blueberries or 1 red Portion Pot® (115g) raspberries

OR

Ⓢ 1 pouch Solo Slim® Low-Fat Beef Meatballs and Potato served with a large mixed salad tossed in oil-free dressing or 200g boiled vegetables (excluding potatoes). Plus 2 satsumas

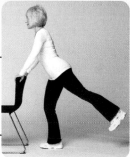

> **Daily fitness challenge**
> Do 40 minutes of aerobic exercise (class or DVD). Do 2 sets of 10 standing back leg lifts.

Day 11

Breakfast

 2 Weetabix served with milk from allowance plus 1 tsp sugar and 10 seedless grapes

OR

 1 × 150g pot 2% fat Greek yogurt served with 100g each raspberries and strawberries plus 50g chopped pineapple and 1 chopped kiwi fruit

Mid-morning Power Snack

 25g low-fat mature cheese (max. 5% fat) plus 2 celery sticks

Lunch

 50g low-fat cottage cheese (any flavour) served with 2 slices wholegrain bread spread with Marmite

OR

200g low-fat cottage cheese served with a large salad tossed in oil-free dressing

OR

 1 pouch Solo Slim® Low-Fat Pea and Mint Soup served with 1 small wholemeal pitta bread or small bread roll

Mid-afternoon Power Snack

1 cereal bowlful of salad

Dinner

 150g lean lamb steak (raw weight), grilled, served with 115g new potatoes (boiled in skins) plus 200g additional vegetables, a little low-fat gravy and mint sauce

OR

 200g lean lamb steak (raw weight), grilled, served with 250g vegetables (excluding potatoes) plus a little low-fat gravy and mint sauce

OR

 Swiss Chard Lasagne (see recipe page 257) served with a large side salad

OR

 150g lean lamb steak, grilled, served with 200g fresh vegetables (excluding potatoes) plus a little low-fat gravy and mint sauce. Plus 1 Müllerlight banana and custard yogurt or other low-fat dessert (max. 100 kcal and 5% fat)

OR

 1 pouch Solo Slim® Low-Fat Lamb Hotpot plus 200g fresh vegetables (excluding potatoes). Plus 1 piece fresh fruit

---

Daily fitness challenge
Walk briskly for 30 minutes. Walk up and down stairs 4 times consecutively.
Do 3 sets of 8 tummy curls (with knees bent).

Day 12

Breakfast

 Tomato and mushrooms on toast: Boil 400g tinned chopped tomatoes until well reduced and season with freshly ground black pepper. Serve on 1 slice toasted wholegrain bread with 10 grilled mushrooms

OR

1 well-grilled rasher lean bacon served with 1 egg, poached, scrambled or dry-fried, 100g grilled mushrooms and 100g tinned tomatoes boiled until reduced

Mid-morning Power Snack

 1 blue Portion Pot® (14g) Special K cereal eaten dry like crisps or served with milk from daily allowance

Lunch

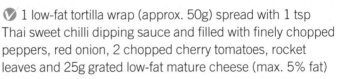 1 low-fat tortilla wrap (approx. 50g) spread with 1 tsp Thai sweet chilli dipping sauce and filled with finely chopped peppers, red onion, 2 chopped cherry tomatoes, rocket leaves and 25g grated low-fat mature cheese (max. 5% fat)

OR

100g cooked chicken breast (no skin), sliced, served with unlimited cos or romaine lettuce plus additional salad, drizzled with 2 dsp low-fat Caesar dressing then topped with 30g grated or shaved low-fat mature cheese (max. 5% fat)

OR

 1 pouch Solo Slim® Low-Fat Carrot and Coriander Soup served with 1 small wholemeal pitta bread or small whole-grain bread roll (max. 150 kcal). Plus 100g fresh fruit salad

Mid-afternoon Power Snack

 1 grilled turkey rasher served with 1 grilled large tomato

Dinner

C Seared Tuna with Chilli Cream (see recipe page 245) served with 150g dry-roasted potatoes and unlimited vegetables or salad. Plus 1 low-fat yogurt (max. 75 kcal and 5% fat)

OR

P Seared Tuna with Chilli Cream (as above recipe) served with and unlimited vegetables (excluding potatoes) or salad. Plus 1 low-fat yogurt (max. 200 kcal and 5% fat)

OR

V Roasted Vegetable Pasta With Garlic Bread (see recipe page 260) served with a small salad tossed in oil-free dressing

OR

D Seared Tuna with Chilli Cream (as above recipe) served with 200g fresh green vegetables. Plus 1 scoop Wall's Soft Scoop Light Ice Cream topped with 100g sliced strawberries

OR

S V 1 pouch Solo Slim® Low-Fat Butternut Squash Soup plus 1 pouch Solo Slim® Low-Fat Three Bean Casserole served with a large mixed salad

Daily fitness challenge
Do 30 minutes of aerobic exercise (brisk walk/jog, bike ride, class or DVD). Do 2 sets of 8 semi press-ups (with knees bent).

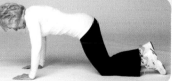
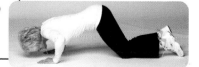

Day 13

Breakfast

 1 red Portion Pot® (40g) Special K Red Berries served with milk from allowance plus 100g fresh fruit

OR

 1 grilled turkey rasher or 1 Quorn Bacon Style Rasher, grilled, served with 1 yellow Portion Pot® (115g) baked beans, plus 6 grilled cherry tomatoes and 50g grilled mushrooms

Mid-morning Power Snack

 150g sliced fresh strawberries

Lunch

 50g low-fat mature cheese (max. 5% fat) on 1 slice wholegrain bread, sprinkled with Worcestershire sauce and then toasted, served with 1 small cereal bowlful salad

OR

50g low-fat mature cheese (max. 5% fat) served with 75g pastrami plus a large mixed salad and 1 dsp extra-light mayonnaise

OR

1 pouch Solo Slim® Low-Fat Pork Meatballs with Smokey Beans served with a large salad tossed in oil-free dressing

Mid-afternoon Power Snack

 1 Hartley's Low Sugar Jelly (max. 10 kcal) plus 1 yellow Portion Pot® (70g) blueberries

Dinner

 Basil and Tomato Cheese Stuffed Chicken (see recipe page 213) served with 100g baby new potatoes (boiled in skins) and a mixed salad

OR

 Basil and Tomato Cheese Stuffed Chicken (as above recipe) served with 200g fresh vegetables of your choice (excluding potatoes)

OR

 Vegetable Biryani (see recipe page 253)

OR

 Basil and Tomato Cheese Stuffed Chicken (as above recipe) served with a large mixed salad. Plus 1 meringue basket filled with 2 tsp 0% fat Greek yogurt and topped with 25g sliced strawberries

OR

(S) 1 pouch Solo Slim® Low-Fat Lentil Soup plus 1 pouch Solo Slim® Low-Fat Chicken Hotpot

Daily fitness challenge
Walk briskly for 40 minutes. Do 2 sets of 8 twisting waist curls.

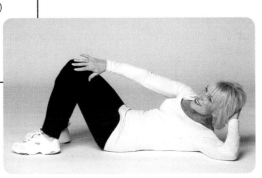

Day 14

Breakfast

Ⓒ ✅ 1 red Portion Pot® (50g) bran flakes or any high-fibre cereal with milk from allowance and 50g fresh strawberries

OR

Ⓟ 2 turkey rashers, grilled or dry-fried, served with 200g tinned tomatoes boiled until reduced, 1 small egg, poached, scrambled or dry-fried and 100g grilled mushrooms

Mid-morning Power Snack

Ⓥ 100g melon plus 1 red Portion Pot® (115g) fresh berries

Lunch

Ⓒ 4 Ryvitas spread with 50g extra-light soft cheese and 50g smoked or tinned salmon, plus sliced cucumber and sprinkled with fresh dill or chives

OR

Ⓟ 100g smoked or tinned salmon served with a large mixed salad tossed in oil-free dressing. Plus 1 blue Portion Pot® (80g) 0% fat Greek yogurt topped with 2 sliced strawberries

OR

Ⓢ ✅ 1 pouch Solo Slim® Low-Fat Mushroom Soup served with 1 small multigrain roll (max. 150 kcal) spread with mustard and filled with 30g wafer thin ham, chicken, beef, turkey or Quorn Deli Ham or Chicken Style Slices

Mid-afternoon Power Snack

 Carrot and sultana salad: 100g grated carrot mixed with 10 sultanas and tossed in oil-free dressing

Dinner

(C) Spicy Mexican Beef (see recipe page 198) served with 1 blue Portion Pot® (55g dry weight) boiled basmati rice

OR

(P) Stir-fry beef: Cut 175g rump steak into strips and stir-fry with 1 dsp reduced-salt soy sauce, 1 dsp sweet chilli sauce and 1 tsp chopped fresh ginger for 3–4 minutes, then add 200g stir-fry vegetables and cook for 3–4 minutes more before serving with additional sweet chilli sauce

OR

(V) Vegetable fajitas (serves 2): Dry-fry 1 sliced red onion, 1 sliced red and green pepper, 1 sliced courgette and 200g sliced mushrooms with a little spray oil and mix with 1 dsp fajita seasoning. Serve each portion in a low-fat tortilla wrap with 1 blue Portion Pot® (75g) tomato salsa per person and a fresh green salad

OR

(D) 100g roast beef served with 200g vegetables of your choice (excluding potatoes) and a little gravy made without fat. Plus 1 × 25g slice fat-free Swiss roll served with 50g low-fat custard

OR

(S) 1 pouch Solo Slim® Low-Fat Beef Goulash served with 100g new potatoes (boiled in skins) and unlimited vegetables (excluding potatoes)

Daily fitness challenge
Do 30 consecutive minutes of energetic housework, gardening or car cleaning.
Go for a 20-minute brisk walk or bike ride.

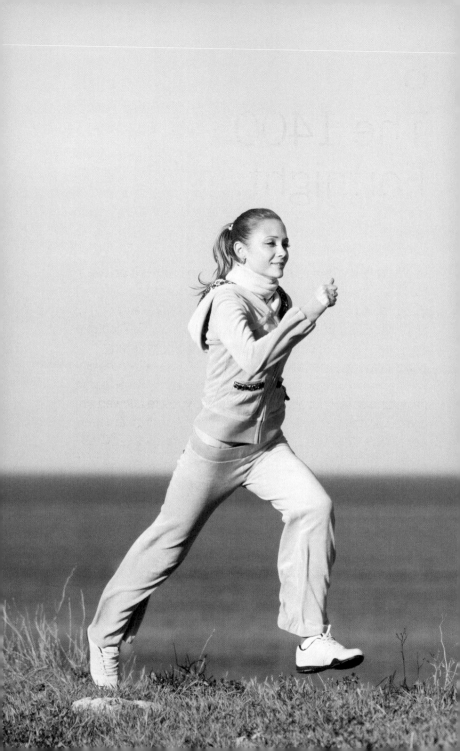

6
The 1400 Fortnight

In weeks three and four, your daily allowance is increased by 200 calories a day to 1400. This means on top of your three main meals and two Power Snacks, you can enjoy an alcoholic drink or high-fat treat each day up to 100 calories. Your high-fat treat can be anything you like, including chocolate or crisps (see page 180 for ideas). Alternatively, you can save up your treat and alcohol calories over seven days for a social occasion. In addition, you are allowed an extra 100 calories a day for a low-fat dessert or treat (see page 181). And should you want to enjoy a large (250ml) glass of wine, that's fine as long as you forgo your treats and dessert for that day.

- **C** = Carbohydrate-based meal
- **P** = High-protein meal
- **V** = Vegetarian meal (or vegetarian option available)
- **S** = Solo Slim® meal

Daily calorie allowance

Breakfast	200 kcal
Mid-morning Power Snack	50 kcal
Lunch	300 kcal
Mid-afternoon Power Snack	50 kcal
Dinner	400 kcal
450ml (¾ pint) skimmed or semi-skimmed milk	approx. 200 kcal

Add-ons for Weeks 3 and 4

Alcoholic drink or high-fat treat	100 kcal
PLUS Low-fat treat or dessert	100 kcal
OR 2 alcoholic drinks or large (250ml) glass wine	200 kcal
Total	**1400 kcal**

Quick guide to alcohol calories

1 yellow Portion Pot (125ml glass) medium white wine	93 kcal
1 yellow Portion Pot (125ml glass) medium red wine	85 kcal
300ml (½ pint) bitter	91 kcal
300ml (½ pint) lager	82 kcal
25ml measure gin/vodka/whisky/rum (use low-cal mixers)	50 kcal

For a more detailed guide to alcohol calories, see page 183.

Weeks 3 & 4:
The 1400 Fortnight

Diet notes

- Spare calories (from unused treats or alcohol) can be saved up over seven days and used for a social occasion.
- The Power Snacks can be eaten mid-morning and mid-afternoon, as suggested, or at another time of day if you prefer.
- You can eat your main meal at lunchtime if you prefer.
- All meals are interchangeable within each category throughout the entire diet.
- You can repeat a meal on subsequent days if you wish, or you can select a meal from the menus in Chapter 8. When making your choices, aim to incorporate five portions of fruit and/or vegetables each day.
- I recommend you continue taking a multivitamin supplement each day to make sure you are getting all the micronutrients for good health.

Free calories

Water, low-cal drinks and tea and coffee (using milk from allowance) are unrestricted.

Day 15

Breakfast

 1 yellow Portion Pot® (14 minis) Weetabix Minis Fruit & Nut, plus 10 seedless grapes and milk from allowance

OR

 2-egg omelette (using milk from allowance), dry-fried and filled with 25g low-fat mature cheese (max. 5% fat) and 4 cherry tomatoes

Mid-morning Power Snack

 1 small apple or pear

Lunch

Cheese, Bacon and Tomato Panini (see recipe page 211)

OR

100g chopped cooked chicken breast or 200g low-fat cottage cheese served with a large mixed salad, topped with 2 dsp low-fat Caesar dressing and sprinkled with 1 tsp parmesan shavings

OR

1 pouch Solo Slim® Low-Fat Tomato and Chilli Risotto. Plus small salad or 1 meringue basket topped with 2 sliced strawberries

Mid-afternoon Power Snack

 100g raw carrots plus 5 cherry tomatoes

Dinner

 85g fresh salmon, grilled, steamed or microwaved, served with 1 blue Portion Pot® (50g uncooked weight) couscous and 100g green vegetables

OR

(P) 115g fresh salmon, grilled, steamed or microwaved, served with 1 yellow Portion Pot® (70g) frozen peas, 200g additional green vegetables and 1 dsp extra-light mayonnaise

OR

 Leek, Broccoli and Cauliflower Cheese (see recipe page 277) served with 2 Quorn sausages, plus a small green salad and 2 grilled tomatoes

OR

 1 pouch Solo Slim® Low-Fat Beef Bolognese plus a large mixed salad tossed in oil-free dressing. Plus 1 piece fresh fruit

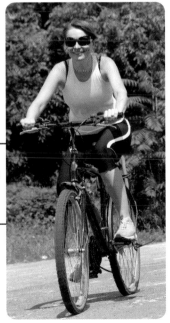

Daily fitness challenge
Do 40 minutes of aerobic exercise (brisk walk/jog, bike ride, class or DVD).

Day 16

Breakfast

 Fruit smoothie: Blend 150g fresh fruit (peaches, strawberries, raspberries or blueberries) with 100g 2% fat Greek yogurt plus milk from allowance

OR

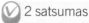 Breakfast yogurt (prepare the night before): 150g 2% fat Greek yogurt mixed with 1 tsp raw oats and 10 sultanas

Mid-morning Power Snack

 2 satsumas

Lunch

 1 slice toasted wholegrain bread topped with 1 × 205g tin baked beans plus 10 cherry tomatoes, grilled

OR

 200g baked beans topped with 1 dry-fried egg and 10 grilled cherry tomatoes

OR

 1 pouch Solo Slim® Low-Fat Tomato Soup. Plus 1 low-fat yogurt (max. 130 kcal and 5% fat)

Mid-afternoon Power Snack

10 cherry tomatoes sprinkled with basil and a little balsamic vinegar

Dinner

 Minced Beef Steaks (see recipe page 191) served with 175g new potatoes (boiled in skins) plus 1 grilled tomato and unlimited additional vegetables

OR

 Minced Beef Steaks (as above recipe but increase beef mince to 400g) served with 200g fresh vegetables of your choice (excluding potatoes)

OR

 100g Quorn Roast Style Sliced Fillets served with 100g dry-roast sweet potatoes plus unlimited spring cabbage and broccoli and a little low-fat gravy

OR

 1 pouch Solo Slim® Low-Fat Carrot and Coriander Soup plus 1 pouch Solo Slim® Low-Fat Beef Bolognese

Daily fitness challenge
Take a 30-minute very brisk walk or bike ride. Do 3 sets of 8 tummy curls (with knees bent).

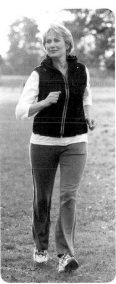

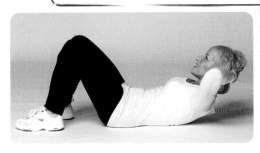

Day 17

Breakfast

 1 slice wholegrain bread, toasted, topped with 1 yellow Portion Pot® (115g) baked beans

OR

 1 egg, scrambled with milk from allowance, served with 75g smoked salmon

Mid-morning Power Snack

 1 fun-size mini banana

Lunch

 1 bagel spread with 40g extra-light soft cheese and topped with 1 sliced tomato and shredded fresh basil leaves

OR

 115g cooked ham, chicken or turkey served with salad. Plus 1 low-fat yogurt (max. 100 kcal and 5% fat)

OR

 1 pouch Solo Slim® Low-Fat Chilli and Rice served on a bed of fresh beansprouts, watercress and sliced tomato

Mid-afternoon Power Snack

Carrot and sultana salad: 100g grated carrot mixed with 10 sultanas and tossed in oil-free dressing

Dinner

 Fennel Jerk Chicken (see recipe page 218) served with 1 blue Portion Pot® (55g dry weight) boiled basmati rice plus unlimited vegetables (excluding potatoes) or salad

OR

 150g chicken breast (no skin) dry-fried with 100g sliced mushrooms and topped with ½ × 295g tin Campbell's Condensed Low Fat Mushroom Soup. Serve with 200g boiled carrots and green vegetables

OR

 Goan Quorn Curry (see recipe page 268) served with 1 blue Portion Pot® (55g dry weight) boiled basmati rice plus a large mixed salad

OR

(S) 1 pouch Solo Slim® Low-Fat Chicken Hotpot served with 200g boiled green vegetables and carrots. Plus 150g fresh fruit salad

Daily fitness challenge
Do 40 minutes of energetic chores such as housework, car cleaning or gardening.

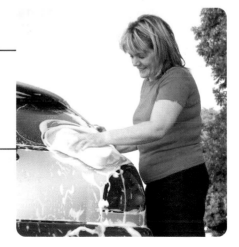

Day 18

Breakfast

 1 green Portion Pot® (40g) Sugar Puffs served with milk from allowance plus 100g fresh fruit

OR

1 grilled turkey rasher or 1 Quorn Bacon Style Rasher, grilled, served with 1 yellow Portion Pot® (115g) baked beans, plus 6 grilled cherry tomatoes and 50g grilled mushrooms

Mid-morning Power Snack

 1 small apple or pear

Lunch

 1 wholegrain roll, halved, spread with extra-light mayonnaise and filled with 50g tinned tuna (in brine or spring water) or low-fat mature cheese (max. 5% fat) plus sliced cucumber

OR

Large salad served with 1 × 100g salmon steak and 2 tsp extra-light mayonnaise

OR

1 pouch Solo Slim® Low-Fat Mushroom Soup. Plus 1 Solo Slim® Nutrition Bar

Mid-afternoon Power Snack

 1 kiwi fruit plus 5 grapes

Dinner

 Barbecue Pork Slices (see recipe page 205) served with 1 small (150g) baked sweet potato and additional fresh vegetables

OR

 Barbecue Pork Slices (see recipe page 205) served with 1 blue Portion Pot® (75g) tomato salsa plus unlimited fresh vegetables (excluding potatoes) or a large mixed salad. Plus 100g fresh fruit salad

OR

 Leek, Broccoli and Cauliflower Cheese (see recipe page 277) served with 2 Quorn sausages, grilled, plus a small green salad and 2 grilled tomatoes

OR

(S) 1 pouch Solo Slim® Low-Fat Beef Goulash served with 100g new potatoes (boiled in skins), plus 100g broccoli and 100g carrots

Daily fitness challenge
Walk up and down stairs 5 times consecutively.
Do 3 sets of 6 semi press ups.
Do 4 sets of 8 tummy curls (with knees bent).

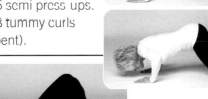

Day 19

Breakfast

 200g fresh fruit salad topped with 100g 2% fat Greek yogurt

OR

 115g cooked lean ham and 1 dry-fried egg

Mid-morning Power Snack

 12 seedless grapes

Lunch

 Tomato, Basil and Cheese Tarts (see recipe page 271) served with a large mixed salad tossed in oil-free dressing

OR

 185g tin tuna (in brine or spring water), drained, served with a large mixed salad tossed in oil-free dressing and topped with ½ hard-boiled egg

OR

 1 pouch Solo Slim® Low-Fat Spicy Beef and Tomato Soup plus 1 small wholegrain roll (max. 150 kcal)

Mid-afternoon Power Snack

1 cereal bowlful of salad

Dinner

 Honey and Mustard Chicken (see recipe page 220) served with 115g boiled new potatoes (with skins) and a mixed salad

OR

 Honey and Mustard Chicken (as above recipe) served with a large mixed salad, no potatoes. Plus 100g fresh fruit salad topped with 1 dsp 2% fat Greek yogurt

OR

Ⓥ Vegetable stir-fry (serves 2): Cook 1 × 350g pack stir-fry vegetables in a preheated non-stick pan with 1 dsp Thai sweet chilli dipping sauce, and serve with 1 blue Portion Pot (55g dry weight) boiled basmati rice per person. Plus 1 low-fat yogurt (max. 100 kcal and 5% fat)

OR

Ⓢ 1 pouch Solo Slim® Low-Fat Chicken Hotpot plus 100g broccoli and 100g cabbage or carrots. Plus 1 low-fat yogurt (max. 100 kcal and 5% fat)

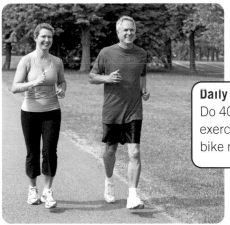

Daily fitness challenge
Do 40 minutes of aerobic exercise (brisk walk/jog, bike ride, class or DVD).

Day 20

Breakfast

 1 slice toasted wholegrain bread spread with Marmite and topped with 50g low-fat mature cheese (max. 5% fat) and 1 sliced tomato, grilled

OR

 3 low-fat pork, beef or Quorn sausages, grilled, served with 2 grilled halved tomatoes

Mid-morning Power Snack

 150g fresh fruit salad

Lunch

Prawn sandwich: 50g prawns mixed with low-fat salad dressing and made into a sandwich with 2 slices wholegrain bread and chopped salad leaves

OR

 100g prawns stir-fried with ½ pack stir-fry vegetables and 1 dsp Thai sweet chilli sauce, served with a little soy sauce. Plus 1 apple or pear

OR

1 pouch Solo Slim® Low-Fat Carrot and Coriander Soup, or similar tinned or fresh soup (max. 80 kcal and 5% fat) with 1 small wholegrain roll (max. 150 kcal); plus 100g fresh fruit salad

Mid-afternoon Power Snack

 1 brown Ryvita or rice cake spread with 20g extra light soft cheese and topped with 2 cherry tomatoes or 2 slices cucumber or chopped chives

Dinner

 Steak and Kidney Pie (see recipe page 195) served with 150g carrots and broccoli

OR

 Steak and Kidney Pie (as above recipe, but exclude potatoes) served with 250g boiled green vegetables. Plus 1 low-fat yogurt (max. 100 kcal and 5% fat)

OR

 Aubergine and Artichoke Gratin (see recipe page 251) served with 100g boiled new potatoes and a large salad. Plus 1 meringue basket topped with 50g strawberries or raspberries and 2 tsp 0% fat Greek yogurt

OR

(S) (V) 1 pouch Solo Slim® Low-Fat Chunky Vegetable Soup plus 1 pouch Solo Slim® Low-Fat Mushroom Stroganoff served with 200g boiled green vegetables

Daily fitness challenge
Take a brisk
30-minute walk.
Stand up and sit down
from a dining chair 8
times, then rest and
repeat 2 more sets.

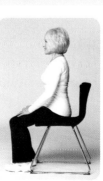
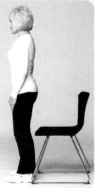

Day 21

Breakfast

 1 blue Portion Pot® (40g) muesli or 40g Fruit 'n Fibre mixed with 100g Total 0% Greek yogurt

OR

150g low-fat wholegrain yogurt (e.g. Onken), any flavour, served with 100g fresh fruit salad

Mid-morning Power Snack

2 satsumas

Lunch

 50g sardines in tomato mashed with 1 tsp extra-light mayonnaise and spread on an open granary bread roll then topped with salad

OR

115g sardines in tomato sauce served with a large salad and extra-light mayonnaise plus ½ hard-boiled egg

OR

 1 pouch Solo Slim® Low-Fat Minestrone Soup or similar (max. 150 kcal and 5% fat) plus 1 Solo Slim® Nutrition Bar and 100g fresh fruit salad

Mid-afternoon Power Snack

 25g low-fat mature cheese (max. 5% fat) plus 2 celery sticks

Dinner

 100g roast beef served with 1 mini Yorkshire pudding, 200g vegetables (excluding potatoes), 50g dry-roasted sweet potatoes and low-fat gravy

OR

 150g roast beef served with 200g vegetables (excluding potatoes) and low-fat gravy

OR

 100g Quorn Roast Style Sliced Fillets served with 100g dry-roast sweet potatoes plus unlimited spring cabbage and broccoli and a little low-fat gravy

OR

 1 pouch Solo Slim® Low-Fat Carrot and Coriander Soup plus 1 pouch Solo Slim® Low-Fat Beef Meatballs and Potato

Daily fitness challenge
Take 2 × 20 minute brisk walks during the day.
Do 3 sets of 6 semi press-ups (with knees bent).

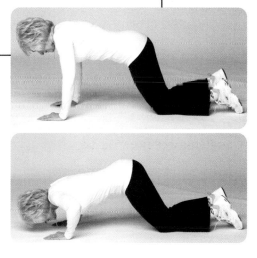

Day 22

Breakfast

 1 slice toasted wholegrain bread topped with 1 poached or dry-fried egg. Plus 1 yellow Portion Pot® (125ml) tomato juice

OR

 2 boiled eggs, plus 200g mixed chopped melon

Mid-morning Power Snack

 1 kiwi fruit plus 6 grapes

Lunch

 1 × 200g jacket potato served with 1 yellow Portion Pot® (115g) baked beans and a large salad

OR

 200g low-fat cottage cheese served with a large salad tossed in oil-free dressing

OR

 1 pouch Solo Slim® Low-Fat Moroccan Spiced Chickpea Tagine. Plus 1 piece fresh fruit

Mid-afternoon Power Snack

 100g raw carrots plus 5 cherry tomatoes

Dinner

 Red Pepper Houmous Baked Cod (see recipe page 248) served with 200g new potatoes (boiled in skins) and unlimited green vegetables

OR

 Red Pepper Houmous Baked Cod (see recipe page 248) served with unlimited fresh vegetables (excluding potatoes). Plus 1 low-fat yogurt (max. 100 kcal and 5% fat)

OR

 Baby Courgette Pasta (see recipe page 263) served with a large salad. Plus 1 low-fat yogurt (max. 100 kcal and 5% fat)

OR

1 pouch Solo Slim® Low-Fat Thai Chicken Curry served with a large mixed salad tossed in oil-free dressing and 1 mini pitta bread

Daily fitness challenge
Do 40 minutes of energetic chores (housework or gardening) or an outdoor family activity such as a bike ride or playing football.

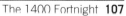

Day 23

Breakfast

 1 Solo Slim® Nutrition Bar plus 1 yellow Portion Pot® (125ml) fresh fruit juice and 1 small apple or pear

OR

 3 low-fat pork, beef or Quorn sausages, grilled, served with 2 grilled halved tomatoes

Mid-morning Power Snack

 150g fresh fruit salad

Lunch

1 wholemeal pitta bread filled with 50g cooked, shelled prawns mixed with 1 dsp low-fat salad dressing, plus chopped tomatoes, celery, peppers and cucumber

OR

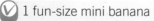 175g tuna steak, grilled, drizzled with balsamic glaze and served with a large salad. Plus 1 small piece fresh fruit

OR

 1 pouch Solo Slim® Low-Fat Vegetable Curry served with 1 blue Portion Pot® (55g dry weight) boiled basmati rice

Mid-afternoon Power Snack

1 fun-size mini banana

Dinner

 Spicy Baked Chicken with Parsnips (see recipe page 222) served with 100g boiled carrots and 100g boiled green vegetables plus 100g new potatoes (boiled in skins)

OR

 Spicy Baked Chicken with Parsnips (as above recipe) served with 300g any vegetables (excluding potatoes). Plus 1 piece fresh fruit

OR

 Chilli Bean Soup (see recipe page 187) served with a large salad and 1 granary bread roll or small baguette

OR

 1 pouch Solo Slim® Low-Fat Chicken Hotpot. Plus 1 Solo Slim® Nutrition Bar

Daily fitness challenge
Walk briskly for 30 minutes. Walk up and down stairs 4 times consecutively.

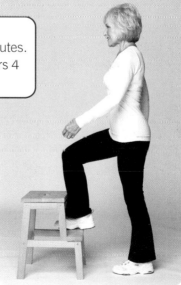

Day 24

Breakfast

 1 small banana, sliced and served with 75g sliced strawberries plus 1 low-fat yogurt (max. 75 kcal and 5% fat)

OR

2 eggs, scrambled with milk from allowance, plus 100g grilled sliced mushrooms and 200g tinned tomatoes boiled until reduced

Mid-morning Power Snack

½ Solo Slim® Nutrition Bar or 1 small apple or pear

Lunch

 Cauliflower and Spinach Soup (see recipe page 186) served with 1 granary roll (max. 150 kcal). Plus 75g fresh fruit salad

OR

100g prawns stir-fried with ½ pack stir-fry vegetables and 1 dsp Thai sweet chilli sauce, served with a little soy sauce. Plus 1 apple or pear

OR

 1 pouch Solo Slim® Low-Fat Chicken and Mushroom Risotto served with a small green salad tossed in oil-free dressing

Mid-afternoon Power Snack

½ Solo Slim® Nutrition Bar or 2 satsumas

Dinner

 Beef and Beer Stew (see recipe page 197) served with 1 small (150g) baked potato plus 200g green vegetables

OR

 Beef and Beer Stew (as above recipe) served with 250g green vegetables and carrots. Plus 1 piece fresh fruit

OR

 Any low-fat vegetarian ready meal or pizza (max. 5% fat and 400 kcal including accompaniments)

OR

(S) 1 pouch Solo Slim® Low-Fat Sausage Casserole served with 200g fresh vegetables (excluding potatoes)

Daily fitness challenge
Do 40 minutes of aerobic exercise (brisk walk/jog, bike ride class or DVD).

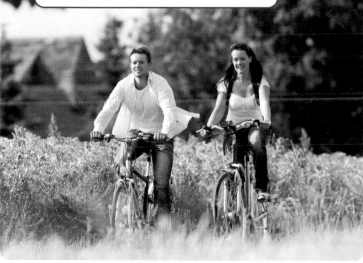

Day 25

Breakfast

 2 Shredded Wheat served with milk from allowance plus 1 dsp strawberries or blueberries and 1 tsp sugar

OR

150g low-fat wholegrain yogurt (e.g. Onken), any flavour, served with 100g fresh fruit salad

Mid-morning Power Snack

90g blueberries

Lunch

100g tinned tuna (in brine or spring water), drained, served with 1 wholemeal pitta bread plus salad and 1 dsp low-fat salad dressing

OR

 100g tinned tuna (in brine or spring water), drained, served with small mixed salad tossed in oil-free dressing, plus 1 blue Portion Pot® (80g) low-fat fruit yogurt and 1 red Portion Pot® (115g) raspberries

OR

1 pouch Solo Slim® Low-Fat Tomato Soup or any other soup of your choice (max. 100 kcal and 5% fat) served with a small multigrain bread roll (max. 150 kcal)

Mid-afternoon Power Snack

1 low-fat yogurt (max. 50 kcal and 5% fat)

Dinner

 Oven-Baked Chicken Tikka Masala (see recipe page 219) served with 50g (cooked weight) boiled basmati rice

OR

 Oven-Baked Chicken Tikka Masala (as above recipe) served with a large mixed salad tossed in oil-free dressing

OR

 Sweet Potato and Fruit Curry (see recipe page 276) served with 1 low-fat mini naan bread plus 1 low-fat yogurt (max. 70 kcal and 5% fat)

OR

 100g cooked chicken tikka breast fillets served with 1 pouch Solo Slim® Low-Fat Spicy Vegetable and Lentil Dhal

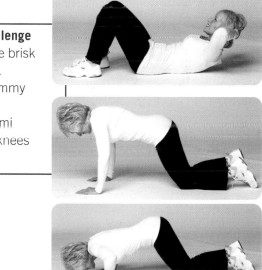

Daily fitness challenge
Take a 45-minute brisk walk or bike ride.
Do 4 sets of 8 tummy curls.
Do 4 sets of 6 semi press-ups (with knees bent).

Day 26

Breakfast

 2 grilled turkey rashers or 2 Quorn Bacon Style Rashers served on 1 slice toasted multigrain bread spread with 1 dsp tomato or brown sauce and topped with 2 grilled tomatoes

OR

(P) 2 grilled turkey rashers served with 1 boiled, poached or dry-fried egg and 1 yellow Portion Pot® (115g) baked beans

Mid-morning Power Snack

(V) 1 kiwi fruit plus 6 grapes

Lunch

 Cheese and apple wrap: Grate 30g low-fat mature cheese (max. 5% fat), ½ apple and 1 small carrot and mix with 1 dsp extra-ight mayonnaise. Serve in a low-fat tortilla wrap

OR

(P) (V) 50g low-fat mature cheese (max. 5% fat), chopped into chunks, served with 1 chopped apple mixed with 50g chopped pineapple and 100g low-fat cottage cheese plus a large salad

OR

(S) (V) 1 pouch Solo Slim® Low-Fat Pea and Mint Soup. Plus 1 Solo Slim® Nutrition Bar and 1 piece fresh fruit

Mid-afternoon Power Snack

 100g raw carrots plus 5 cherry tomatoes

Dinner

 Pork and Red Pepper Burgers (see recipe page 204) served with 1 × 200g baked sweet potato plus a large salad and 1 blue Portion Pot® (75g) tomato salsa

OR

 Pork and Red Pepper Burgers (as above recipe) served with a large salad and 1 blue Portion Pot® (75g) tomato salsa. Plus 1 low-fat yogurt or fromage frais (max. 150 kcal and 5% fat)

OR

 1 vegetarian burger (max. 180 kcal and 5% fat) served with 175g new potatoes (boiled in skins), plus 1 grilled tomato and unlimited additional vegetables

OR

(S) 1 pouch Solo Slim® Low-Fat Carrot and Coriander Soup, plus 1 pouch Solo Slim® Low-Fat Beef Meatballs and Potato

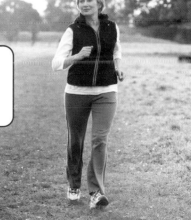

Daily fitness challenge
Do 40 minutes of aerobic exercise (brisk walk/jog, bike ride, class or DVD).

Day 27

Breakfast

 1 blue Portion Pot® (35g dry weight) porridge oats, made up and cooked with water, served with milk from allowance, 1 tsp runny honey, 15g sultanas or raisins and a sprinkling of cinnamon

OR

P 115g cooked lean ham and 1 dry-fried egg

Mid-morning Power Snack

200g fresh melon

Lunch

C BLT sandwich: Toast 2 slices wholegrain bread, spread 1 slice with 1 tsp extra-light mayonnaise and the other with 1 tsp tomato ketchup and fill with 25g lean grilled bacon, 1 slice wafer-thin chicken, lettuce leaves and 1 sliced tomato

OR

 2 low-fat beef, pork or Quorn sausages, grilled, served with 1 yellow Portion Pot® (115g) baked beans, plus 1 × 200g tomatoes boiled until reduced and unlimited grilled or boiled mushrooms

OR

 1 pouch Solo Slim® Low-Fat Tomato and Vegetable Pasta served with a large mixed salad

Mid-afternoon Power Snack

 1 low-fat yogurt (max. 50 kcal and 5% fat)

Dinner

 Roast Turkey Leg Fricassee (see recipe page 229) served with 40g (dry weight) boiled basmati rice

OR

 Roast Turkey Leg Fricassee (as above recipe) served with 200g fresh vegetables of your choice (excluding potatoes)

OR

 Watercress and Tomato Pasta (see recipe page 278) topped with 30g grated low-fat mature cheese (max. 5% fat) and served with a large mixed salad tossed in oil-free dressing. Plus 1 piece fresh fruit

OR

(S) 1 pouch Solo Slim® Low-Fat Thai Chicken Curry plus either 200g stir-fried vegetables or 1 pouch Solo Slim® Low-Fat Mushroom Soup

Daily fitness challenge
Do 30 minutes of aerobic exercise (brisk walk/jog, bike ride, class or DVD).
Stand up and sit down 8 times, then rest and repeat 3 more sets.

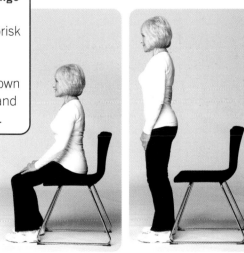

Day 28

Breakfast

 1 yellow Portion Pot® (40g) any low-fat muesli (max. 5% fat) served with milk from allowance and 1 tsp sugar

OR

 1 low-fat beef or pork sausage (max. 5% fat), grilled, plus 1 well-grilled lean bacon rasher served with 2 tomatoes, halved and grilled, and 1 dry-fried egg

Mid-morning Power Snack

 200g fresh melon

Lunch

 1 yellow Portion Pot® (45g dry weight) pasta shapes, boiled with a vegetable stock cube, drained and mixed with ½ × 340g jar (170g) low-fat tomato and basil pasta sauce, heated through

OR

 115g thin-cut lean beef steak dry-fried with 300g stir-fry vegetables and a little soy sauce

OR

 1 pouch Solo Slim® Low-Fat Spicy Mixed Bean Soup. Plus 1 Solo Slim® Nutrition Bar

Mid-afternoon Power Snack

12 cherry tomatoes

Dinner

 Apple-Stuffed Pork Fillet (see recipe page 206) served with 150g new potatoes (boiled in skins) or 1 yellow Portion Pot® cooked sweet potato plus 100g carrots and 100g broccoli

OR

 Apple-Stuffed Pork Fillet (as above recipe) served with 300g boiled vegetables (excluding potatoes). Plus 1 blue Portion Pot® (80g) 2% fat Greek yogurt mixed with 1 red Portion Pot® (115g) raspberries

OR

Any ready-made vegetarian bake (max. 200 kcal and 5% fat) served with 150g new potatoes (boiled in skins) and unlimited other vegetables and salad

OR

1 pouch Solo Slim® Low-Fat Lentil Soup plus 1 pouch Solo Slim® Low-Fat Lamb Hotpot

---

Daily fitness challenge

Do 45 minutes of aerobic exercise (brisk walk/jog, bike ride, class or DVD).
Walk up and down stairs 5 times consecutively.

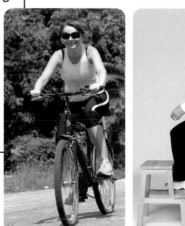

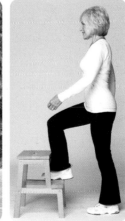

7
Your Personal FAB Plan

If you have completed the first four weeks of my FAB Diet, well done! You should have lost a significant amount of weight and inches and be looking and feeling slimmer and fitter.

You can now move on to part three: Your Personal FAB Plan. To find your personal daily calorie allowance, check the charts on pages 360–61, looking at the figure in the column against your gender, age and current weight. This figure is equivalent to your basal metabolic rate (BMR), which is the number of calories you burn in keeping your blood circulating, organs working and your body renewing and repairing itself in any 24-hour period. As soon as you start moving around and going about your everyday activities and doing some physical exercise, you will be using extra calories and burning fat from your body's fat stores. At every 1-stone loss, you should reduce your personal calorie allowance to ensure that your rate of weight loss progresses as swiftly and healthily as possible until you reach your ultimate goal.

What to eat

It's likely you'll have extra calories to spend on healthy foods of your choice over and above the 1200 calories in the basic diet, unless you are aged over 60 or are only slightly overweight.

You can choose any breakfast, lunch, dinner and Power Snacks from the daily diet menus and the suggestions in Chapter 8. All the breakfasts are 200 calories, lunches are 300 calories, dinners 400 calories and Power Snacks 50 calories each. Always remember to use your daily milk allowance of 450ml (¾ pint) milk (200 calories) and this will take you up to your basic 1200 calories. I also recommend you keep taking a multivitamin supplement each day just to be sure that you are getting all the necessary micronutrients for good health.

If you have extra calories available, you can use these for a low-fat dessert or treat and if your calorie allowance permits, you can enjoy an alcoholic drink or a high-fat treat up to 100 calories. If your calorie allowance is 1200 or less, but you'd like to enjoy a glass of wine occasionally, that's fine but make sure you do an additional 30 minutes of exercise that day to burn the extra calories.

I realise that shift workers can find it difficult to stick to a regular eating plan, so I have given some general guidelines along with a sample diet menu plan on pages 126–8.

Fat Loss Booster Day

If your calorie allowance is more than 1200, choose one day a week as your Fat Loss Booster Day in order to give your weight loss a further boost. On that day, stick to 1200 calories (as in the Kick-Start Booster Diet) with no alcohol or treats and do 30 minutes of fairly energetic exercise. You can choose any day of the week you like – whatever suits your schedule and lifestyle. For instance, Monday might be a good day after a sociable weekend, or you might prefer another day in the week when you're likely to be really busy – though you'll need to find time to exercise – and won't want to have an alcoholic drink.

Make the diet fit your lifestyle

If you don't drink alcohol, you can use your calories elsewhere. If you want to drink 2 glasses of wine and not have a treat, you can. If you don't fancy a dessert that day, you can add an extra portion of rice, pasta or potatoes to your main meal. It's this flexibility of choice that will enable you to achieve long-term success.

If you have a lot of weight to lose

If you have a lot of weight to lose and your personal calorie allowance is, say 1800, then rather than using your 'extra' calories on alcohol and treats, it would be preferable to increase your portions of rice, pasta, potatoes or cereals at meal times. Remember to weigh your portions or use your Portion Pots® for accuracy.

Boost your fitness

Once you've completed the daily fitness challenges in the first four weeks, you can take your fitness and fat-burning to a whole new level by committing to follow the Advanced FAB Fitness Challenge in Chapter 12. I also recommend you continue with the Five-Minute Core Workout in Chapter 11.

Week 5 onwards: Your Personal FAB Plan

Daily allowance

Breakfast	200 kcal
Mid-morning Power Snack	50 kcal
Lunch	300 kcal
Mid-afternoon Power Snack	50 kcal
Dinner	400 kcal
450ml (¾ pint) skimmed or semi-skimmed milk	approx. 200 kcal
Total	**1200 kcal**

Extras (depending on your calorie allowance)
- 1 alcoholic drink or high-fat treat per day (max. 100 kcal)
- 1 low fat dessert or low fat treat per day (max. 100 kcal)
- Extra portions of rice, cereal, potatoes, etc. (see below)

Extra calorie suggestions
If your personal calorie allowance permits you can add extra foods to the meal suggestions in this book by mixing or matching these ideas to meet your daily allowance.

Approx. 50 calories extra
Breakfast
- 28g portion of high-fibre cereal, e.g. All-Bran, Fruit 'n Fibre
- 55g portion of baked beans
- 2 grilled turkey rashers
- 1 piece fresh fruit (excluding bananas)

- 1 Weetabix
- 1 Shredded Wheat
- 150ml unsweetened fruit juice
- 12 seedless grapes

Lunch
- Add an extra 75g portion of boiled new potatoes
- Increase portion of rice by 15g uncooked weight or 35g cooked weight
- Increase portion of pasta by 15g uncooked weight or 40g cooked weight
- 55g whole prawns

Dinner
- Add an extra 75g portion of boiled new potatoes
- Add a large mixed salad with fat-free dressing
- 120ml any clear or vegetable soup
- 1 measure of spirits, e.g. gin, vodka, whisky, with a low-calorie mixer
- 1 piece extra fresh fruit

Approx. 100 calories extra
Breakfast
- 28g muesli with extra fruit
- 1 slice wholegrain bread
- 1 pot low-fat yogurt (max. 100 kcal and 5% fat)
- 1 large banana
- 1 large egg, poached, boiled or dry-fried

Lunch
- 1 slice wholegrain bread

- Add an extra 150g portion of boiled new potatoes
- Increase rice portion by 28g dry weight or 70g cooked weight
- Increase pasta portion by 28g dry weight or 85g cooked weight
- 1 blue Portion Pot® (100g) low-fat cottage cheese
- 1 pouch Solo Slim® Low-Fat Carrot and Coriander Soup
- 4 grilled turkey rashers
- 2 pieces fresh fruit
- 1 large banana
- 100ml fruit sorbet
- 55g ready-to-eat dried apricots or prunes

Dinner
- Have 1 pouch Solo Slim® Low-Fat Carrot and Coriander Soup as a starter
- Increase portion of red meat by 40g
- Increase portion of poultry by 55g
- Increase portion of fish by 85g
- Increase rice portion by 28g dry weight or 70g cooked weight
- Increase pasta portion by 28g dry weight or 85g cooked weight
- Add an extra 150g portion of boiled new potatoes
- 1 × 150ml glass wine
- 300ml (½ pint) lager

Approx. 150 calories extra
Breakfast
- 1 blue Portion Pot® (40g) muesli
- 1 red Portion Pot® (40g) Special K
- 1 green Portion Pot® (40g) Sugar Puffs

Approx. 150 calories extra (continued)

Lunch
- 1 medium slice toasted wholegrain bread spread with 2 tsp marmalade or preserve
- 2 medium bananas
- 3 extra pieces of fresh fruit (excluding bananas)
- 1 Solo Slim® soup (max. 150 kcal)
- 85g lean grilled chicken breast (no skin, weighed without bone)
- 85g lean grilled fillet steak

Dinner
- Any combination of 1×50 kcal and 1×100 kcal suggestions
- Have a Solo Slim® soup (max. 150 kcal) as a starter
- 85g lean grilled chicken breast (no skin, weighed without bone)
- 85g lean grilled fillet steak
- 2 meringue nests filled with 55g chopped fruit and topped with 1 tbsp low-fat yogurt
- 1 pot low-fat yogurt (max. 150 calories and 5% fat)
- 55g raisins

A sample menu plan for shift workers

If you work shifts it's best to think of your diet in 'one-week' chunks rather than in days. For instance, if your personal daily calorie allowance is 1500, then over a week you should consume 10,500 calories. A shift worker needs to have six meals a day, which will in effect include two breakfasts. So, have breakfast before you go to bed and then have another, higher-calorie breakfast when you get up. Eat your two 'Power Snacks' when it suits you best and have your main meal to fit in with your shift pattern. Enjoy an alcoholic drink if you wish. Then you will still have your alcohol/treat/dessert calories to use when you choose.

Daily diet plan

Over a 24-hour period on a 1500 calories per day allowance, your menu plan could look like this (based on a 1500-calorie allowance):

Daily allowance

450ml (¾ pint) semi-skimmed milk   200 kcal

Breakfast 1 (before bed)
Ⓥ 2 Shredded Wheat served with milk from allowance plus 1 dsp blueberries and 1 tsp sugar 200 kcal

Breakfast 2 (on rising)
Ⓟ Ⓥ 2 well-grilled rashers lean bacon or veggie alternative, served with 1 medium egg, dry-fried or poached, and 1 × 200g tin tomatoes boiled until reduced   200 kcal
Plus 1 slice toasted wholegrain bread   100 kcal

Main meal
Ⓟ 115g thin-cut lean beef steak dry-fried with 300g stir-fry vegetables and a little soy sauce   400 kcal

Alcohol
1 small glass wine   100 kcal

Treat
1 small (21.9g) Milky Way   98 kcal

Dessert
1 low-fat yogurt (max. 5% fat)   100 kcal

Power Snacks (2 per day)
2 satsumas   50 kcal

PLUS 1 rice cake spread with 20g extra light soft
cheese (max. 5% fat) and 2 slices cucumber   50 kcal

When the weight won't budge

When you start a diet, you are likely to see a fast weight loss early on. Hopefully, on my FAB Diet you will have continued to lose weight and made fantastic progress. But when you've been following a diet plan for a number of weeks, you may find that your weight stalls and the scales just seem not to want to cooperate.

Sandra wrote to me in desperation, explaining: 'I have the diet book, I go to classes every week, I only buy low-fat foods and I exercise at least three times a week, yet some weeks nothing seems to be happening. What else can I do?' I meet people like Sandra at my own classes – and I have met lots of 'Sandras' over the years. I've been there myself. I can remember being obsessed with trying to lose weight and the harder I tried, the more it seemed to pile on. So I know how Sandra is feeling.

The problem is that the more obsessed you become about losing weight, the more you think about food. What shall I have for breakfast? Lunch? Tonight? And the more you think about food, the hungrier you become. It's inevitable as food is at the forefront of your mind, so you need to change that thought pattern. You can do this by planning ahead for the week rather than making meal decisions when you are hungry.

Here are my top 10 ways to give your weight loss a boost:

1 Plan your menu for the week and stick to it. Include some of your favourite recipes or dishes from the diet plan. Avoid buying anything extra, no matter how good the supermarket offers are this week. Having made your plan, switch off from thinking about food. It's sorted.

2 Check your portion sizes. Weigh your food or use your Portion Pots® to measure your servings of rice, pasta, breakfast cereal. Having too big a portion size is the number one reason why we don't lose weight when we're trying to stick to a diet plan.

3 Keep a food diary (or blog). This will help you focus on your achievements. It's not all about what the scales say, so try to reflect on the changes you have made to your diet, and note down any benefits you've noticed – such as feeling less breathless, or a compliment someone has paid you. If you find yourself facing a difficult situation, think about how you coped and whether there is anything different you could do next time. In quiet moments turn to your diary instead of a snack.

4 Wear your pedometer. It will motivate you to walk more as you try to reach a new target.

5 Each day, record what you eat and how many steps you take. Reflect on your progress and look for changes over time to spot those areas where you aren't sticking to the plan quite so carefully.

6 Stay busy so you're not tempted to snack. How many times do you find yourself nibbling an extra snack in the evening when you finally sit down to relax and enjoy the first quiet moments of the day? Keeping busy – by doing something you enjoy that is different from your usual routine – can be both relaxing and diverting, leaving no time for a snack. If you persist in snacking – other than having your 'Power Snacks' – you are unlikely to succeed on your weight-loss plan.

7 Don't buy anything that might tempt you in a weak moment. Buying fun-size chocolate bars and bumper bags of crisps in case the children bring their friends around is a poor excuse and you will only end up eating them.

8 When preparing your meals keep a careful eye on the quantities of the food you are cooking. We all hate waste, so we end up dividing the contents of the colander, that last slice of meat or portion of pasta or rice on to our plates. That's where you run the risk of seriously jeopardising your progress.

9 Leave those leftovers alone. If you can't face scraping the plates into the bin, get someone else to do it for you.

10 Watch your alcohol consumption. Drinking alcohol is a habit and can weaken our willpower. One drink can easily lead to another…

The golden rule is that if you're not losing weight you're eating too many calories and not exercising enough. Correct these and I guarantee you'll start to lose weight at a steady rate again. Trust me – it works!

8
Diet menus

Choose any breakfast, lunch and dinner, plus a couple of 'power snacks' a day from the following lists. All the breakfasts are 200 calories, all lunches 300 calories, all dinners 400 calories and all 'power snacks' 50 calories. In addition, you can select a high-fat treat or alcoholic drink (max. 100 kcal), plus a low-fat treat or low-fat dessert (max. 100 kcal) each day if your calorie allowance permits. If you have extra calories to spend see pages 123–6 for ideas.

Breakfasts   132
Lunches   140
Dinners   155
Power Snacks   177
Treats and Desserts   180
Alcoholic Drinks   183

= Carbohydrate-based meal

= High-protein meal

= Vegetarian meal (or vegetarian option available)

= Dinner with a dessert

= Solo Slim® meal

Breakfasts

Cereal breakfasts (approx. 200 kcal each)

- 1 blue Portion Pot® (35g dry weight) porridge oats, cooked with water and served with milk from allowance plus 1 tsp honey and 1 kiwi fruit
- 1 blue Portion Pot® (35g dry weight) porridge oats, made up and cooked with water, served with milk from allowance, 1 tsp runny honey, 15g sultanas or raisins and a sprinkling of cinnamon
- Creamy muesli (serves 1; prepare the night before): Mix ½ blue Portion Pot® (20g) muesli with 1 blue Portion Pot® (80g) 2% fat Greek yogurt and a little milk from allowance (enough to make the consistency of a thick cream) and leave overnight. To serve, add more milk if necessary plus 1 small tsp runny honey and 1 small banana, sliced
- Energy muesli (serves 1; prepare the night before): Mix 15g dry porridge oats, 10g sultanas, 4 chopped almonds, 1 coarsely grated apple, 1 coarsely grated carrot with 50g low-fat natural yogurt. Serve with additional milk from allowance if required
- 1 blue Portion Pot® (40g) muesli (max. 5% fat) or 40g Fruit 'n Fibre mixed with 100g 0% fat Greek yogurt
- 1 blue Portion Pot® (40g) low-fat muesli (max. 5% fat) served with milk from allowance plus 100g sliced strawberries
- 1 yellow Portion Pot® (50g) any low-fat muesli (max. 5% fat) served with milk from allowance and 1 tsp sugar

✔ 1 blue Portion Pot® (80g) low-fat yogurt (any flavour) topped with 1 blue Portion Pot® (40g) low-fat muesli (max. 5% fat) and 2 sliced strawberries

✔ Soak 15g All-Bran overnight in 100g low-fat natural yogurt with 4 chopped almonds, 10 sultanas and 1 tsp honey. Serve with a little milk from allowance if required

✔ 1 red Portion Pot® (50g) any bran cereal (e.g. Sultana Bran, All-Bran, bran flakes) served with milk from allowance plus 1 tsp sugar or 1 sliced small apple

✔ 1 yellow Portion Pot® (25g) Sultana Bran or other bran cereal served with milk from allowance. Plus 1 yellow Portion Pot® (125ml) unsweetened fruit juice

✔ 1 red Portion Pot® (50g) bran flakes or any high-fibre cereal served with milk from allowance and 50g sliced fresh strawberries

✔ 1 yellow Portion Pot® (125ml) unsweetened pure orange juice. Plus 1 red Portion Pot® (40g) Special K cereal served with milk from allowance and 1 tsp sugar

✔ 1 red Portion Pot® (30g) Sugar Puffs served with milk from allowance and 1 pot low-fat yogurt, any flavour (max. 80 kcal and 5% fat)

✔ 2 Shredded Wheat served with milk from allowance plus 1 dsp blueberries and 1 tsp sugar

✔ 2 Weetabix served with milk from allowance plus 1 tsp sugar and 10 seedless grapes

✔ 2 Weetabix served with milk from allowance and 1 yellow Portion Pot® (70g) blueberries mixed with 1 red Portion Pot® (115g) raspberries

✔ 1 red Portion Pot® (35g) Weetabix Weetos served with milk from allowance and 100g fresh fruit salad

⊘ 1 yellow Portion Pot® (14 minis) Weetabix Minis Fruit & Nut, plus 10 seedless grapes and milk from allowance

⊘ 1 red Portion Pot® (35g) Special K Red Berries cereal served with milk from allowance plus 100g fresh fruit

⊘ 1 yellow Portion Pot® (34g) Nestlé Coco Shreddies served with milk from allowance plus 1 yellow Portion Pot® (125ml) fruit juice

⊘ 1 red Portion Pot® (43g) Kellogg's Coco Pops Choc 'n' Roll cereal served with milk from allowance and 100g melon

⊘ 1 yellow Portion Pot® (30g) Special K Peach & Apricot cereal served with milk from allowance and 1 sliced fresh peach

Fruit and yogurt breakfasts (approx. 200 kcal each)

⊘ 1 small banana plus 1 × 180ml pack Innocent Fruit Smoothie (any flavour)

⊘ 2 bananas

⊘ 1 small banana, sliced and served with 75g sliced strawberries plus 1 low-fat yogurt (max. 75 kcal and 5% fat)

⊘ 1 low-fat yogurt (max. 100 kcal and 5% fat) mixed with 1 sliced large banana

⊘ Fruit smoothie (serves 1): Blend 150g fresh fruit (peaches, strawberries, raspberries or blueberries) with 100g 2% fat Greek yogurt plus milk from allowance

⊘ Medley of melon, strawberries and raspberries (200g total) topped with 50g 0% fat Greek yogurt

☑ 200g fresh fruit salad topped with 100g 2% fat Greek yogurt

☑ 250g tropical fruit salad (chopped melon, pineapple, mango, papaya and kiwi) topped with 1 blue Portion Pot® (80g) 2% fat Greek yogurt

P

☑ Breakfast yogurt (serves 1; prepare the night before): 150g 2% fat Greek yogurt mixed with 1 tsp raw oats and 10 sultanas

☑ 150g low-fat wholegrain yogurt (e.g. Onken), any flavour, served with 100g fresh fruit salad

☑ 1 × 150g pot 2% fat Greek yogurt served with 100g each raspberries and strawberries plus 50g chopped pineapple and 1 chopped kiwi fruit

☑ 2 Müllerlight yogurts, any flavour

☑ 200g 2% fat Greek yogurt served with 100g fresh strawberries, blueberries or raspberries

Quick and easy carbohydrate breakfasts

(approx. 200 kcal each)

C

☑ 1 slice wholegrain toast spread with 2 tsp marmalade, jam or honey. Plus ½ grapefruit sprinkled with granulated sweetener

☑ 1 slice wholegrain bread, toasted, spread with 2 tsp marmalade, jam or honey. Plus 200g tropical fruit salad (sliced melon, mango and pineapple)

☑ 1 low-fat cereal bar (max. 100 kcal and 5% fat) plus 1 large banana

☑ 1 Solo Slim® Nutrition Bar (any flavour) plus 100g sliced strawberries with 50g 0% fat Greek yogurt

✅ 1 crumpet spread with 1 blue Portion Pot® (80g) 2% fat Greek yogurt and topped with 1 red Portion Pot® (115g) fresh raspberries

✅ 1 crumpet, toasted, spread with 1 tsp jam, marmalade or honey and served with 1 pot low-fat yogurt (max. 75 kcal and 5% fat)

✅ 1 crumpet, toasted, topped with 2 dsp 2% fat Greek yogurt, 1 tsp strawberry or raspberry jam and 50g sliced strawberries

✅ 1 yellow Portion Pot® (125ml) fresh orange juice. Plus 1 boiled egg and 1 wholegrain Ryvita crispbread spread with Marmite (optional)

✅ 1 slice toasted wholegrain bread spread with Marmite if desired and topped with 1 poached or dry-fried egg. Plus 1 yellow Portion Pot® (125ml) fresh orange or tomato juice

✅ 1 egg, boiled, poached or scrambled, served on 1 slice toasted wholegrain bread. Plus 100g tinned grapefruit (in juice) or ½ fresh grapefruit sprinkled with 1 tsp granulated sweetener

Cooked carbohydrate breakfasts (approx. 200 kcal each)

• 1 slice toasted wholegrain bread topped with 200g tinned tomatoes boiled until reduced, plus 2 grilled turkey rashers

✅ 1 slice toasted wholegrain bread topped with 1 yellow Portion Pot® (115g) baked beans

✅ 1 boiled or poached egg served on 1 slice toasted wholegrain bread spread with Marmite if desired. Plus 125ml fresh orange juice

Ⓒ ✅ 1 egg, boiled, poached or scrambled, served on 1 slice toasted wholegrain bread. Plus 100g tinned grapefruit (in juice) or ½ fresh grapefruit sprinkled with 1 tsp granulated sweetener

✅ 1 egg, poached, boiled or scrambled, served on 1 slice toasted wholegrain bread, plus 1 large tomato, halved and grilled

• 1 crumpet, toasted, topped with 20g extra-light soft cheese, served with 1 grilled turkey rasher and 100g grilled mushrooms

✅ 1 egg, boiled or poached, served on 1 slice wholegrain bread, toasted and spread with Marmite. Plus 200g melon

✅ Tomato and mushrooms on toast: Boil 400g tinned chopped tomatoes until well reduced and then season with freshly ground black pepper. Serve on 1 slice toasted wholegrain bread with 10 grilled mushrooms

Strawberry muesli

High-protein cooked breakfasts (approx. 200 kcal each)

(P)

- 1 low-fat beef or pork sausage (max. 5% fat), grilled, served with 1 poached or scrambled egg plus 100g mushrooms, sliced and dry-fried, and 200g tinned tomatoes boiled until reduced
- 2 low-fat pork or beef sausages, grilled, served with 2 large tomatoes, halved and grilled, and 50g grilled or dry-fried mushrooms
- 2 grilled turkey rashers served with 1 dry-fried or scrambled egg, 100g sliced mushrooms and 200g tinned tomatoes boiled until reduced
- 4 grilled turkey rashers served with 1 yellow Portion Pot® (115g) baked beans and 2 grilled tomatoes
- 2 grilled turkey rashers served with 1 large grilled tomato and 50g sliced mushrooms, grilled or dry-fried, plus 1 yellow Portion Pot® (115g) baked beans
- 1 egg, poached or dry-fried, served with 2 grilled turkey rashers and unlimited grilled tomatoes and mushrooms
- 1 well-grilled rasher lean bacon served with 1 egg, poached, scrambled or dry-fried, 100g grilled mushrooms and 100g tinned tomatoes boiled until reduced
- 2 well-grilled rashers lean bacon served with 1 small egg, dry-fried or poached, and 100g tinned tomatoes boiled until reduced
- 1 egg, boiled or poached, served with 75g wafer-thin ham and 1 tomato, sliced. Plus ½ grapefruit sprinkled with granulated sweetener if required
- 60g smoked salmon served with 1 large scrambled egg made using milk from allowance

(P) • 1 low-fat beef or pork sausage (max. 5% fat), grilled, plus 1 rasher lean bacon, well grilled, served with unlimited fresh tomatoes, halved and grilled, and 1 small egg, poached, scrambled or dry-fried
• 2-egg omelette (made using milk from allowance) dry-fried and filled with 50g sliced mushrooms and 20g wafer-thin ham
• 115g cooked lean ham and 1 dry-fried egg

High-protein vegetarian cooked breakfasts
(approx. 200 kcal each)

(P) ✓ 2 eggs, scrambled, dry-fried or poached, plus 3 tomatoes, halved and grilled, and 50g mushrooms, grilled or dry-fried
✓ 1 Quorn Bacon Style Rasher, grilled, served with 1 yellow Portion Pot® (115g) baked beans, plus 6 grilled cherry tomatoes and 50g grilled mushrooms
✓ 3 Quorn sausages, grilled, served with 2 grilled halved tomatoes
✓ 2 Quorn sausages, grilled, served with 1 egg, dry-fried or poached, and 200g tinned tomatoes boiled until reduced
✓ 2 Quorn sausages, grilled, served with unlimited grilled mushrooms and fresh tomatoes
✓ 1 Quorn Bacon Style Rasher served with 1 yellow Portion Pot® (115g) baked beans plus 1 tomato, halved and grilled, and 50g grilled mushrooms

Lunches

Soup lunches (approx. 300 kcal each)

ⓒ ⓥ Chilli Bean Soup (see recipe page 187) served with a large salad and 1 granary bread roll or small baguette

ⓥ Cauliflower and Spinach Soup (see recipe page 186) served with 1 granary roll (max. 150 kcal). Plus 75g fresh fruit salad

ⓥ Sweet Potato and Leek Soup (see recipe page 188) served with 1 small wholegrain bread roll (max. 150 kcal)

ⓥ Roasted Aubergine, Pepper and Chilli Soup (see recipe page 189) served with 1 small wholegrain bread roll (max. 150 kcal). Plus 1 pot low-fat yogurt (max. 70 kcal and 5% fat)

Sandwich snack lunches: meat, chicken and turkey
(approx. 300 kcal each)

ⓒ • 2 slices wholegrain bread spread with low-fat salad dressing and filled with 50g wafer-thin chicken or ham or beef, plus 1 sliced tomato, unlimited salad leaves, sliced cucumber and chopped celery

• Cheese, Bacon and Tomato Panini (see recipe page 211)

• BLT sandwich: Toast 2 slices wholegrain bread, spread 1 slice with 1 tsp extra-light mayonnaise and the other with 1 tsp tomato ketchup and fill with 25g lean grilled bacon, 1 slice wafer-thin chicken, lettuce leaves and 1 sliced tomato

- 2 slices wholegrain bread spread with HP Fruity Sauce then filled with 3 grilled turkey rashers and sliced tomatoes
- 2 slices wholegrain bread or 1 small wholegrain bread roll spread with mustard, pickle or extra-light mayonnaise and filled with 50g wafer-thin ham, turkey or chicken plus salad
- 1 slice wholegrain bread spread with extra-light mayonnaise and made into an open sandwich with 100g cooked pastrami, pickled gherkins and salad
- 1 small wholegrain bread roll (max. 150 kcal), halved, spread with mustard, pickle or extra-light mayonnaise and made into open sandwiches with 100g cooked chicken breast, salad leaves, sliced spring onions and cucumber
- 1 mini pitta bread filled with 50g wafer-thin ham or chicken and salad with 1 tsp low-fat salad dressing. Plus 1 bag Ryvita minis (any flavour)
- 1 low-fat tortilla wrap (approx. 50g) spread with 1 tsp Thai sweet chilli dipping sauce and filled with finely chopped peppers, red onion, 2 chopped cherry tomatoes, rocket leaves and 25g chopped chicken (no skin)

Sandwich lunches: fish and seafood

(approx. 300 kcal each)

- 2 slices wholegrain bread filled with 50g prawns mixed with low-fat salad dressing and chopped salad leaves
- 50g sardines in tomato mashed with 1 tsp extra-light mayonnaise then spread on an open granary bread roll (max. 150 kcal) and topped with salad

(C)

- 1 small wholegrain bread roll (max. 150 kcal) spread with 25g extra-light soft cheese and filled with 25g smoked salmon, plus a small salad
- 1 wholegrain bread roll (max. 150 kcal), halved, spread with extra-light mayonnaise and filled with 50g tinned tuna (in brine or spring water) plus sliced cucumber
- 1 large wholemeal pitta bread filled with unlimited salad plus 50g cooked shelled prawns and drizzled with 1 dsp Thai sweet chilli dipping sauce
- 1 medium wholemeal pitta bread filled with 50g cooked shelled prawns mixed with 1 dsp low-fat salad dressing, plus chopped tomatoes, celery, peppers and cucumber
- 1 medium wholemeal pitta bread filled with 100g tinned tuna (in brine or spring water), drained and mixed with 1 dsp low-fat salad dressing, plus salad vegetables
- 1 low-fat tortilla wrap spread with 1 dsp Thai sweet chilli dipping sauce and filled with either 50g tinned tuna (in brine or spring water) or 50g cooked shelled prawns plus chopped salad vegetables (e.g. peppers, celery, spring onions, cherry tomatoes, cucumber) and shredded rocket leaves
- 1 medium wholemeal pitta bread filled with low-calorie seafood dressing, rocket leaves and 100g cooked shelled prawns or 25g low-fat mature cheese (max. 5% fat) or 50g low-fat cottage cheese (any flavour)
- Smoked Mackerel Pâté (see recipe page 233) served with 1 toasted wholemeal pitta bread (max. 135 kcal)

• 4 Ryvitas spread with 50g extra-light soft cheese and 50g smoked or tinned salmon, plus sliced cucumber and sprinkled with fresh dill or chives

Sandwich lunches: vegetarian (approx. 300 kcal each)

✓ 2 thin slices wholegrain bread spread with extra-light mayonnaise, mustard, pickle or horseradish and filled with 50g Quorn Deli Ham or Chicken Style Slices, plus sliced cucumber, tomato and salad leaves

✓ 2 slices wholegrain bread spread with Marmite and filled with 50g low-fat cottage cheese

✓ 1 slice wholegrain bread topped with 50g low-fat mature cheese (max. 5% fat), sprinkled with Worcestershire sauce, then toasted and served with 1 small cereal bowlful salad

✓ 2 slices wholegrain bread spread with 1 dsp extra-light mayonnaise and filled with 1 sliced hard-boiled egg and salad vegetables

✓ Any ready-made sandwich (max. 300 kcal and 5% fat)

✓ 1 small wholegrain bread roll (max. 150 kcal), halved, spread with pickle or extra-light mayonnaise and made into open sandwiches with 50g low-fat mature cheese (max. 5% fat), salad leaves, sliced spring onions and cucumber

✓ 1 bagel spread with 40g extra-light soft cheese and topped with 1 sliced tomato and shredded fresh basil leaves

✓ 100g low-fat houmous served with 1 wholemeal pitta bread plus 200g carrots, cucumber and celery cut into crudités

✅ 1 low-fat tortilla wrap spread with 1 tsp Thai sweet chilli dipping sauce and filled with finely chopped peppers, red onion, 2 chopped cherry tomatoes, rocket leaves and 25g grated low-fat mature cheese (max. 5% fat)

✅ Cheese and apple wrap (serves 1): Grate 30g low-fat mature cheese (max. 5% fat), ½ apple and 1 small carrot and mix with 1 dsp extra-light mayonnaise. Serve in a low-fat tortilla wrap

✅ 1 medium wholemeal pitta bread filled with low-calorie salad dressing, rocket leaves and 25g low-fat mature cheese (max. 5% fat) or 50g low-fat cottage cheese (any flavour)

✅ 4 Ryvitas or rice cakes topped with 100g low-fat cottage cheese and unlimited salad vegetables

Pasta or rice salad lunches (approx. 300 kcal each)

• Tuna pasta salad (serves 1): Cook 1 yellow Portion Pot® (45g dry weight) pasta shapes in boiling water with a vegetable stock cube. Drain and leave to cool, then mix with 100g tinned tuna (in brine or spring water) plus shredded lettuce, chopped cucumber, tomatoes and spring onions, all tossed in fat-free salad dressing

• Chicken pasta salad (serves 1): Cook 1 yellow Portion Pot® (45g dry weight) pasta shapes in boiling water with a vegetable stock cube. Drain and leave to cool, then mix with unlimited salad vegetables and 50g chopped cooked chicken breast (no skin) all tossed in fat-free salad dressing

© ● 100g tikka-flavoured cooked chicken breast chopped and mixed with 50g (cooked weight) boiled basmati rice, unlimited chopped salad vegetables and 20g sultanas. Add 2 dsp extra-light mayonnaise mixed with 1 tsp mild curry powder and chopped coriander

Ⓥ Quorn pasta salad (serves 1): Cook 1 yellow Portion Pot® (45g dry weight) pasta shapes in boiling water with a vegetable stock cube. Drain and leave to cool, then mix with 100g Quorn Deli Chicken Style Slices, chopped, plus shredded lettuce, chopped cucumber, tomatoes and spring onions all tossed in fat-free salad dressing

Carbohydrate cooked lunches (approx. 300 kcal each)

© ● Smoked Fish Laksa (see recipe page 246) served with 75g crusty wholegrain bread

● Sweet Chilli Prawns (see recipe page 242) served with 1 blue Portion Pot® (55g dry weight) boiled basmati rice

Ⓥ Vegetable Biryani (see recipe page 253). Plus 100g fresh fruit with 1 dsp 0% fat Greek yogurt

Ⓥ 1 egg, poached, boiled or scrambled, served with 1 slice toasted wholegrain bread. Plus 1 small banana and 1 low-fat yogurt (max. 60 kcal and 5% fat)

Ⓥ 1 × 200g baked sweet potato topped with 1 blue Portion Pot® (100g) low-fat cottage cheese (any flavour), plus a small mixed salad tossed in fat-free dressing

Ⓥ 1 × 200g baked sweet or regular potato served with 1 yellow Portion Pot® (115g) baked beans plus a large salad tossed in fat-free dressing

Ⓒ ✓ 1 slice wholegrain bread, toasted, topped with 1 yellow Portion Pot® (115g) baked beans. Plus 1 low-fat yogurt (max. 60 kcal and 5% fat)

✓ 1 slice toasted wholegrain bread topped with 1 × 205g tin baked beans plus 10 cherry tomatoes, grilled

✓ Tomato and Asparagus Pasta (see recipe page 264) served with 1 low-fat chocolate pudding (max. 150 kcal and 5% fat), e.g. Cadbury Light Chocolate Mousse

✓ Tomato and Asparagus Pasta (see recipe page 264). Plus 1 Müllerlight yogurt (any flavour)

✓ Tomato, Basil and Cheese Tarts (see recipe page 271) served with a large mixed salad tossed in oil-free dressing

✓ 1 yellow Portion Pot® (45g dry weight) pasta shapes, boiled with a vegetable stock cube, drained and mixed with ½ × 340g jar (170g) low-fat tomato and basil pasta sauce, heated through

High-protein salad lunches: meat and chicken

(approx. 300 kcal each)

Ⓟ • 2 chicken drumsticks (skin removed) served with a small side salad tossed in oil-free dressing

• 75g pastrami plus 50g low-fat mature cheese (max. 5% fat) served with a large mixed salad and 1 dsp extra-light mayonnaise

• 75g chopped cooked chicken breast mixed with 1 tbsp low-calorie salad dressing and ½ tsp curry powder, then served with a large mixed salad including chopped fruits (e.g. melon, pineapple, strawberries) plus salad vegetables with rocket leaves

- 100g cooked pastrami served with a large mixed salad tossed in oil-free dressing plus 50g mixed pickles. Plus 1 low-fat yogurt (max. 100 kcal and 5% fat)
- 75g wafer-thin ham served with a large mixed salad tossed in oil-free dressing or extra-light mayonnaise. Plus 100g fresh fruit salad
- 150g cooked chicken or turkey breast (no skin), grilled, served with a large mixed salad tossed in oil-free salad dressing
- 100g cooked chicken breast (no skin), sliced, served with unlimited cos or romaine lettuce plus additional salad, drizzled with 2 dsp low-fat Caesar dressing then topped with 30g grated or shaved low-fat mature cheese (max. 5% fat)
- 120g cooked chicken breast (no skin) served with a Waldorf salad: Mix 1 chopped apple, 2 chopped celery sticks, 15g sultanas, 4 chopped walnut halves and shredded lettuce leaves with 1 dsp extra-light mayonnaise and 1 dsp low-fat natural yogurt
- 115g cooked ham, chicken or turkey served with salad. Plus 1 low-fat yogurt (max. 100 kcal and 5% fat)
- 100g cooked chicken breast served with a large salad with low-calorie dressing. Plus 100g strawberries topped with 1 dsp 0% fat Greek yogurt

High-protein salad lunches: fish and seafood
(approx. 300 kcal each)

- 100g tinned tuna (in brine or spring water), drained, served with small mixed salad tossed in oil-free dressing. Plus 1 blue Portion Pot® (80g) low-fat fruit yogurt and 1 red Portion Pot® (115g) raspberries

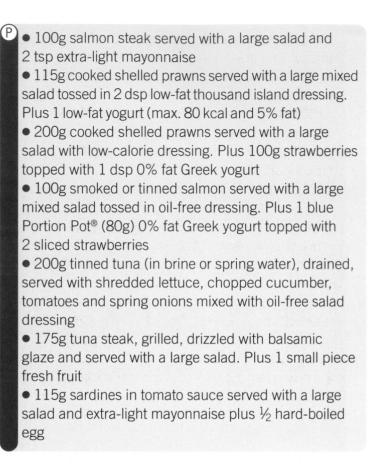

- 100g salmon steak served with a large salad and 2 tsp extra-light mayonnaise
- 115g cooked shelled prawns served with a large mixed salad tossed in 2 dsp low-fat thousand island dressing. Plus 1 low-fat yogurt (max. 80 kcal and 5% fat)
- 200g cooked shelled prawns served with a large salad with low-calorie dressing. Plus 100g strawberries topped with 1 dsp 0% fat Greek yogurt
- 100g smoked or tinned salmon served with a large mixed salad tossed in oil-free dressing. Plus 1 blue Portion Pot® (80g) 0% fat Greek yogurt topped with 2 sliced strawberries
- 200g tinned tuna (in brine or spring water), drained, served with shredded lettuce, chopped cucumber, tomatoes and spring onions mixed with oil-free salad dressing
- 175g tuna steak, grilled, drizzled with balsamic glaze and served with a large salad. Plus 1 small piece fresh fruit
- 115g sardines in tomato sauce served with a large salad and extra-light mayonnaise plus ½ hard-boiled egg

High-protein salad lunches: vegetarian

(approx. 300 kcal each)

- 50g low-fat mature cheese (max. 5% fat) served with 1 small mixed salad tossed in oil-free dressing. Plus 1 low-fat yogurt (max. 100 kcal and 5% fat)
- 2 hard-boiled eggs served with a large mixed salad tossed in oil-free dressing. Plus 1 kiwi fruit and 1 satsuma

⊙ 50g low-fat mature cheese (max. 5% fat), chopped into chunks, served with 1 chopped apple mixed with 50g chopped pineapple and 100g low-fat cottage cheese plus a large salad

⊙ 100g low-fat mature cheese (max. 5% fat) served with a large salad served with low-calorie dressing. Plus 100g strawberries topped with 1 dsp 0% fat Greek yogurt

⊙ 200g low-fat cottage cheese served with a large mixed salad, topped with 2 dsp low-fat Caesar dressing and sprinkled with 1 tsp shaved low-fat mature cheese (max. 5% fat)

⊙ 120g Quorn Deli Chicken Style Slices served with a Waldorf salad: Mix 1 chopped apple, 2 chopped celery sticks, 15g sultanas, 4 chopped walnut halves and shredded lettuce leaves with 1 dsp extra-light mayonnaise and 1 dsp low-fat natural yogurt

⊙ 100g Quorn Deli Chicken Style Slices served with large mixed salad plus 2 dsp low-fat Caesar dressing and topped with 20g shaved low-fat mature cheese (max. 5% fat)

High-protein cooked lunches (approx. 300 kcal each)

● 115g thin-cut lean beef steak dry-fried with 300g stir-fry vegetables and a little soy sauce

● 1 yellow Portion Pot® (115g) baked beans served with 2 well-grilled rashers lean bacon and 50g grilled mushrooms

⊙ 100g cooked chicken breast (no skin) or Quorn Deli Chicken Style Slices served with 200g stir-fry vegetables dry-fried with a little soy sauce. Plus 150g fresh fruit

(P) • 100g shelled prawns stir-fried with ½ pack stir-fry vegetables and 1 dsp Thai sweet chilli sauce, served with a little soy sauce or balsamic vinegar. Plus 1 apple or pear

(V) 2 low-fat beef, pork or Quorn sausages, grilled, served with 1 yellow Portion Pot® (115g) baked beans, plus 200g tinned tomatoes boiled until reduced and unlimited grilled or boiled mushrooms

(V) 200g baked beans topped with 1 dry-fried egg and 10 grilled cherry tomatoes

(V) 2-egg omelette cooked with milk from allowance and filled with 100g sliced mushrooms, spring onions and 20g low-fat cheese (max 5% fat). Serve with a mixed salad tossed in oil-free dressing

Solo Slim® lunches: meat, chicken and fish

(approx. 300 kcal each)

(S) • 1 pouch Solo Slim® Low-Fat Beef Goulash. Plus 1 piece fresh fruit

• 1 pouch Solo Slim® Low-Fat Chilli and Rice served on a bed of fresh beansprouts, watercress and sliced tomato

• 1 pouch Solo Slim® Low-Fat Spicy Beef and Tomato Soup plus 2 Ryvitas spread with extra-light mayonnaise and topped with sliced tomatoes and salad

• 1 pouch Solo Slim® Low-Fat Mushroom Soup plus 1 small wholegrain bread roll (max. 150 kcal) spread with mustard and filled with 30g wafer-thin ham, chicken, beef or turkey

• 1 pouch Solo Slim® Low-Fat Lamb Hotpot plus 100g boiled broccoli

- 1 pouch Solo Slim® Low-Fat Pork Meatballs with Smokey Beans plus a large salad tossed in oil-free dressing
- 1 pouch Solo Slim® Low-Fat Chicken Hotpot
- 1 pouch Solo Slim® Low-Fat Chicken and Mushroom Risotto served with a small green salad tossed in oil-free dressing
- 1 pouch Solo Slim® Low-Fat Chicken and Mushroom Risotto. Plus 1 satsuma or plum
- 1 pouch Solo Slim® Low-Fat Carrot and Coriander Soup, or similar tinned or fresh soup (max. 80 kcal and 5% fat) with large mixed salad tossed in oil-free dressing and 100g wafer-thin ham, turkey, chicken, beef or Quorn Chicken or Ham Deli Slices

Solo Slim® vegetarian lunches (approx. 300 kcal each)

- 1 pouch Solo Slim® Low-Fat Tomato Soup. Plus 1 low-fat yogurt (max. 130 kcal and 5% fat)
- 1 pouch Solo Slim® Low-Fat Leek and Potato Soup. Plus 1 Solo Slim® Nutrition Bar or 100g fresh fruit salad
- 1 pouch Solo Slim® Low-Fat Mushroom Soup. Plus 1 Solo Slim® Nutrition Bar (any flavour) or 100g fresh fruit salad
- 1 pouch Solo Slim® Low-Fat Minestrone Soup plus 1 Solo Slim® Nutrition Bar (any flavour) and 100g fresh fruit salad
- 1 pouch Solo Slim® Low-Fat Minestrone Soup plus 2 Ryvitas spread with 1 tsp very-low-fat mayonnaise and topped with 25g grated low-fat mature cheese (max. 5% fat) and 1 sliced tomato

(S)

✓ 1 pouch Solo Slim® Low-Fat Tomato Soup plus 1 small wholegrain bread roll (max. 150 kcal)

✓ 1 pouch Solo Slim® Low-Fat Chunky Vegetable Soup served with 1 small wholegrain bread roll (max. 150 kcal). Plus 1 satsuma or kiwi fruit

✓ 1 pouch Solo Slim® Low-Fat Spicy Mixed Bean Soup plus 2 Ryvitas spread with extra-light soft cheese and topped with sliced cucumber and tomato

✓ 1 pouch Solo Slim® Low-Fat Spicy Mixed Bean Soup. Plus 1 Solo Slim® Nutrition Bar

✓ 1 pouch Solo Slim® Low-Fat Lentil Soup served with 1 wholemeal pitta bread. Plus 100g fresh fruit salad

✓ 1 pouch Solo Slim® Low-Fat Pea and Mint Soup plus 1 mini wholemeal pitta bread or small bread roll (max. 150 kcal)

✓ 1 pouch Solo Slim® Low-Fat Pea and Mint Soup. Plus 1 Solo Slim® Nutrition Bar and 1 piece fresh fruit

✓ 1 pouch Solo Slim® Low-Fat Carrot and Coriander Soup plus 1 small wholemeal pitta bread or wholegrain bread roll (max. 150 kcal). Plus 100g fresh fruit salad

✓ 1 pouch Solo Slim® Low-Fat Butternut Squash Soup plus 1 small wholegrain bread roll (max. 150 kcal)

✓ 1 pouch Solo Slim® Low-Fat Vegetable Curry. Plus 1 Solo Slim® Nutrition Bar and 1 satsuma or kiwi fruit

✓ 1 pouch Solo Slim® Low-Fat Tomato and Vegetable Pasta served with a large mixed salad

✓ 1 pouch Solo Slim® Low-Fat Vegetable Curry served with 1 blue Portion Pot® (55g dry weight) boiled basmati rice

✓ 1 pouch Solo Slim® Low-Fat Tomato and Chilli Risotto. Plus a small salad or 1 meringue basket topped with 2 sliced strawberries

Ⓢ

Ⓥ 1 pouch Solo Slim® Low-Fat Three Bean Casserole. Plus 1 low-fat yogurt (max. 100 kcal and 5% fat)

Ⓥ 1 pouch Solo Slim® Low-Fat Mushroom Stroganoff plus a large mixed salad or 2 pieces fresh fruit

Ⓥ 1 pouch Solo Slim® Low-Fat Three Bean Casserole served with 1 blue Portion Pot® (55g dry weight) boiled basmati rice

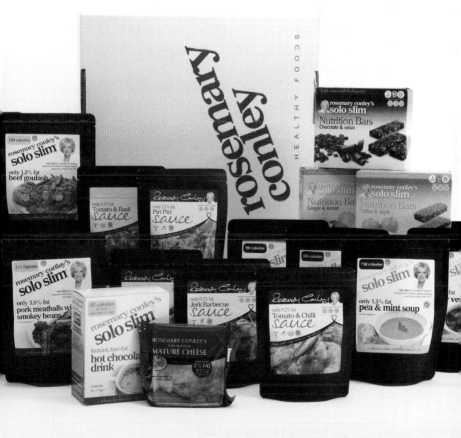

Lunch recipes using Rosemary Conley cooking sauces
(approx. 300 kcal each)

Rosemary Conley Low-Fat Thai Red Sauce:

Ⓒ • Thai Cod Laksa (see recipe page 249) served with
1 × 150g wholegrain bread roll

Ⓟ • Thai Red Chicken Curry (see recipe page 227)
served with a large mixed salad tossed in oil-free
dressing

Rosemary Conley Low-Fat Tomato and Basil Sauce:

Ⓒ • Sausage Penne with Tomato and Basil Sauce (see
recipe page 212)

Rosemary Conley Low-Fat Tomato and Chilli Sauce:

Ⓒ Ⓥ Spicy Tagliatelle with Tomato and Chilli Sauce (see
recipe page 280) served with a large mixed salad
tossed in oil-free dressing

Rosemary Conley Low-Fat Piri Piri Sauce:

Ⓟ • Piri Piri Pork (see recipe page 209) served with a
large mixed salad tossed in oil-free dressing

Ⓒ Ⓥ Spicy Mini Pizza (see recipe page 279) served with
a large mixed salad tossed in oil-free dressing

Dinners

Carbohydrate dinners: beef, lamb and pork

(approx. 400 kcal each)

- 125g lean roast beef or lamb served with 100g dry-roasted sweet potatoes, 200g fresh vegetables of your choice (e.g. carrots, broccoli, cauliflower) and a little low-fat gravy
- 150g lean steak, grilled, served with 1 blue Portion Pot® (75g) tomato salsa plus 115g new potatoes, (boiled in their skins), and a large mixed salad
- 150g lean beef steak, grilled, served with 100g oven chips (max. 5% fat) plus 1 large beef tomato, halved and grilled, 1 dsp tomato ketchup and a large mixed salad
- 2 low-fat beef or pork sausages (max. 5% fat), grilled, served with 1 red Portion Pot® (250g) mashed sweet potato plus 100g spring greens or sliced cabbage, 100g cauliflower or broccoli and a little low-fat gravy
- Spicy Mexican Beef (see recipe page 198) served with 1 blue Portion Pot® (55g dry weight) boiled basmati rice
- Ginger Beef Stir-Fry with Noodles (see recipe page 192) served with 1 dsp sweet chilli sauce
- Minced Beef Steaks (see recipe page 191) served with 175g new potatoes (boiled in their skins) plus 1 grilled tomato and unlimited fresh vegetables (excluding potatoes)
- Beef and Beer Stew (see recipe page 197) served with 1 small (150g) baked potato plus 200g green vegetables

- Steak and Kidney Pie (see recipe page 195) served with 150g carrots and broccoli
- 150g lean lamb steak, grilled, served with 115g new potatoes (boiled in skins) plus 200g fresh vegetables (excluding potatoes), a little low-fat gravy and mint sauce
- 125g lean roast pork served with 125g dry-roasted potatoes, plus 200g fresh vegetables (excluding potatoes) and gravy made without fat
- Black Bean Pork (see recipe page 203) served with 1 blue Portion Pot® (55g dry weight) boiled basmati rice
- Pork and Red Pepper Burgers (see recipe page 204) served with 1 × 200g sweet potato, baked in its skin, plus a large salad and 1 blue Portion Pot® (75g) tomato salsa
- Barbecue Pork Slices (see recipe page 205) served with 1 small (150g) sweet potato, baked in its skin, and unlimited fresh vegetables (excluding potatoes)
- Pork and Leek Casserole (see recipe page 207) served with 1 yellow Portion Pot® (100g) mashed sweet potato and unlimited green vegetables
- Mint Salsa Lamb Steak (see recipe page 201) served with either 1 blue Portion Pot® (50g dry weight) couscous or 200g new potatoes (boiled in skins) plus either a large salad tossed in oil-free dressing or 50g carrots and 50g broccoli
- Apple-Stuffed Pork Fillet (see recipe page 206) served with 150g new potatoes (boiled in skins) or 1 yellow Portion Pot® (100g) cooked sweet potato plus 100g carrots and 100g broccoli

Carbohydrate dinners: chicken and turkey
(approx. 400 kcal each)

- 125g roast chicken or turkey (no skin) served with 125g dry-roasted potatoes, plus 200g fresh vegetables (excluding potatoes) and gravy made without fat
- 1 × 125g chicken breast (no skin), grilled or microwaved, served with 100g each carrots, broccoli and new potatoes (boiled in skins) plus a little low-fat gravy
- Chicken fajita (serves 1): Dry-fry 1 small chicken breast (no skin) with 1 tsp fajita spice mix, ½ sliced onion and ½ sliced red and green pepper. Serve in 1 low-fat (max. 5% fat) tortilla wrap with a large mixed salad and 1 blue Portion Pot® (75g) tomato salsa
- Chicken and mushroom pie (serves 2): Dry-fry 200g chopped skinless chicken breast, then transfer to a pie dish. Add 1 chopped small onion, 150g sliced mushrooms, cover with 1 × 295g tin Campbell's Condensed Low Fat Mushroom Soup and season with plenty of black pepper. Top with 300g cooked mashed potato and bake in the oven at 200°C, 400°F, Gas Mark 6 for 20 minutes. Serve with 200g boiled carrots and green vegetables
- Quick and easy chicken curry (serves 1): Dry-fry 1 × 115g chopped chicken breast (no skin) in a preheated non-stick pan with ½ chopped onion and 1 crushed garlic clove. Sprinkle 1 tsp curry powder over and 'cook out' for 1 minute, then add 1 small chopped chilli, ½ chopped green pepper, 25g button mushrooms (optional) and 400g tinned chopped tomatoes, and simmer for 5 minutes to reduce. Serve with 1 blue Portion Pot® (55g dry weight) boiled basmati rice

- Chicken stir-fry (serves 1): Dry-fry 100g sliced chicken breast (no skin) with 2 crushed garlic cloves in a non-stick pan until the chicken is almost cooked. Add a selection of chopped vegetables (e.g. peppers, onions, carrots, courgettes, celery, beansprouts), plus soy sauce to taste and 2 tsp sweet chilli sauce. When the chicken is cooked through, serve with 1 blue Portion Pot® (55g dry weight) boiled basmati rice
- Honey and Mustard Chicken (see recipe page 220) served with 115g boiled new potatoes (with skins) and a mixed salad
- Cajun Chicken Casserole (see recipe page 216) served with 1 yellow Portion Pot® (100g) mashed sweet potato plus 100g green vegetables
- Fennel Jerk Chicken (see recipe page 218) served with 1 blue Portion Pot® (55g dry weight) boiled basmati rice plus unlimited vegetables (excluding potatoes) or salad
- Chicken Korma (see recipe page 214) served with 1 blue Portion Pot® (55g dry weight) boiled basmati rice
- Oven-Baked Chicken Tikka Masala (see recipe page 219) served with 50g (cooked weight) boiled basmati rice
- Spicy Baked Chicken with Parsnips (see recipe page 222) served with 100g boiled carrots and 100g boiled new potatoes (with skins) plus 100g green vegetables
- Crispy Turkey Escalopes with Noodles (see recipe page 230) served with a large mixed salad
- Roast Turkey Leg Fricassee (see recipe page 229) served with 40g (dry weight) boiled basmati rice
- Turkey Spaghetti (see recipe page 228) served with a large mixed salad and 2 dsp low-fat dressing

Carbohydrate dinners: fish (approx. 400 kcal each)

- 1 rainbow trout, grilled, poached or barbecued with black pepper and lemon juice, served with 115g new potatoes (boiled in skins), 1 yellow Portion Pot® (70g) frozen peas, 100g carrots and 1 dsp extra-light mayonnaise
- 100g salmon steak, grilled, steamed or microwaved, served with 1 blue Portion Pot® (50g dry weight) couscous plus unlimited vegetables or salad and 1 dsp sweet chilli sauce
- 100g salmon steak, grilled, steamed or microwaved, served with 100g new potatoes (boiled in their skins) plus 100g mangetout and 1 tsp Thai sweet chilli dipping sauce mixed with 1 dsp extra-light mayonnaise
- 100g salmon steak, grilled, steamed or microwaved, served with unlimited stir-fried vegetables and a little soy sauce plus 115g new potatoes (boiled in skins)
- 85g fresh salmon, grilled, steamed or microwaved, served with 1 blue Portion Pot® (50g dry weight) couscous and 100g green vegetables
- Salmon Fish Fingers (see recipe page 239) served with Bombay Potatoes (see recipe page 252) and a mixed leaf salad
- Red Pepper Houmous Baked Cod (see recipe page 248) served with 200g new potatoes (boiled in skins) and green vegetables
- Coconut Prawns (see recipe page 244) served with 125g (cooked weight) boiled basmati rice
- Tandoori Salmon with Spicy Noodles (see recipe page 238) served with 100g stir-fry vegetables

Carbohydrate dinners: vegetarian (approx. 400 kcal each)

- 100g Quorn Roast Style Sliced Fillets served with 100g dry-roast sweet potatoes plus unlimited spring cabbage and broccoli and a little low-fat gravy

- 1 low-fat pizza (max. 350 kcal and 5% fat) served with a mixed salad tossed in oil-free dressing

- Sweet and sour vegetable stir-fry: Chop ½ onion, ½ red pepper and 1 celery stick and dry-fry with 50g sliced mushrooms, handful of mangetout and baby corn until soft. Add 125g (1 portion) low-fat sweet and sour sauce. Serve with 1 blue Portion Pot® (55g dry weight) boiled basmati rice and a little soy sauce

- 2 Quorn sausages, grilled, served with 1 red Portion Pot® (250g) mashed sweet potato, plus 100g spring greens or sliced cabbage, 100g cauliflower or broccoli and a little low-fat gravy

- Roasted Vegetable Sausages (see recipe page 272) served with 1 × 200g baked sweet potato

- Crushed Bean Rigatoni (see recipe page 254) served with a large salad. Plus 1 piece fresh fruit

- Roasted Vegetable Pasta with Garlic Bread (see recipe page 260) served with a small salad tossed in oil-free dressing

- Goan Quorn Curry (see recipe page 268) served with 1 blue Portion Pot® (55g dry weight) boiled basmati rice plus a large mixed salad

- Leek, Broccoli and Cauliflower Cheese (see recipe page 277) served with 2 Quorn sausages, grilled, plus a small green salad and 2 grilled tomatoes

- Any low-fat vegetable soup (max. 120 kcal and 5% fat) plus Crushed Bean Rigatoni (see recipe page 254)

✔ Swiss Chard Lasagne (see recipe page 257) served with a large side salad

✔ Vegetable fajitas (serves 2): Dry-fry 1 sliced red onion, 1 sliced red and green pepper, 1 sliced courgette and 200g sliced mushrooms with a little spray oil and mix with 1 dsp fajita seasoning. Serve each portion in a low-fat tortilla wrap with 1 blue Portion Pot® (75g) tomato salsa per person and a fresh green salad

✔ Chilli Bean Soup (see recipe page 187) served with a large salad and 1 granary bread roll or small baguette

✔ 1 vegetarian burger (max. 180 kcal and 5% fat) served with 175g new potatoes (boiled in skins), plus 1 grilled tomato and unlimited additional vegetables

✔ Watercress and Tomato Pasta (see recipe page 278) topped with 30g grated low-fat mature cheese (max. 5% fat) and served with a large mixed salad tossed in oil-free dressing. Plus 1 piece fresh fruit

✔ Any ready-made vegetarian meal (max. 200 kcal and 5% fat) served with 150g new potatoes (boiled in skins) and unlimited other vegetables and salad

✔ Roasted vegetable pasta (serves 2): Roast a selection of sliced vegetables (e.g. 1 red and green pepper, 100g mushrooms, 1 red onion and 1 courgette) in a moderate oven until lightly browned, then mix the vegetables with 1 jar tomato-based pasta sauce and heat through. Serve with 1 yellow Portion Pot® (45g dry weight) pasta shapes per person (boiled with a vegetable stock cube) and sprinkle with 20g grated low-fat mature cheese (max. 5% fat) per person

ⓥ 3 Quorn or other veggie sausages, grilled, served with 1 yellow Portion Pot® mashed sweet potato plus unlimited green vegetables, 1 yellow Portion Pot® (75g) tinned sweetcorn and a little gravy made without fat

ⓥ Cook 1 yellow Portion Pot® (45g dry weight) pasta shapes in boiling water with a vegetable stock cube. Drain and add ½ jar (approx. 200g) ready-made low-fat tomato and basil pasta sauce and heat through. Serve with chopped fresh basil and 1 tbsp 25g grated low-fat mature cheese (max. 5% fat)

ⓥ 1 × 225g baked potato topped with 50g low-fat mature cheese (max. 5% fat) and 1 yellow Portion Pot® (115g) baked beans, served with a small mixed salad

ⓥ Veggie bolognese (serves 1): Dry-fry 100g Quorn mince or similar with chopped peppers, mushrooms, onions and courgettes. Mix in ½ jar low-fat pasta sauce or similar and heat through. Serve with 1 yellow Portion Pot® (45g dry weight) pasta shapes cooked in boiling water with a vegetable stock cube

ⓥ Vegetable curry (serves 2): Mix a selection of unlimited chopped vegetables (onions, peppers, courgettes, mushrooms, cauliflower) with ½ jar of low-fat curry sauce (max. 100 kcal and 5% fat per serving). Serve with 1 blue Portion Pot® (55g dry weight) boiled basmati rice per person

ⓥ Vegetable chilli (serves 1): Mix 1 × 400g tin red kidney beans in chilli sauce with chopped onion, peppers, mushrooms, courgettes, 1 crushed garlic clove and 1 × 400g tin chopped tomatoes. Serve with 1 blue Portion Pot® (55g dry weight) boiled basmati rice and a small side salad

High-protein dinners: beef, lamb and pork

(P) • 175g rump steak, grilled, served with 1 blue Portion Pot® (75g) tomato salsa plus a large mixed salad and 1 tomato, halved and grilled

• 175g lean roast beef or lamb or 200g roast pork served with 200g vegetables (excluding potatoes) of your choice plus a little low-fat gravy

• 120g rump steak, grilled, served with a large mixed salad tossed in oil-free dressing plus 2 tomatoes, halved and grilled. Plus 1 meringue basket topped with 1 blue Portion Pot® (80g) 0% fat Greek yogurt and 1 yellow Portion Pot® (70g) blueberries or 1 red Portion Pot® (115g) raspberries, or any other low-fat dessert of your choice (max. 125 kcal and 5% fat)

• 2 low-fat beef or pork sausages, grilled, served with 1 yellow Portion Pot® (115g) baked beans, 200g tinned tomatoes boiled until reduced plus unlimited grilled or boiled mushrooms

• Minced beef in gravy: Dry-fry 100g extra-lean minced beef in non-stick pan, then remove from pan and drain off all the fat. Add 1 chopped small onion, 1 sliced carrot, 1 sliced courgette and 100g sliced mushrooms to the pan and dry-fry until soft. Season well with black pepper and add the cooked mince. Make up 300ml (½ pint) low-fat gravy with gravy powder and 1 beef stock cube as per packet instructions and pour over the mince mixture. Serve with 100g boiled green vegetables (excluding potatoes)

• Oriental Beef Stir-Fry (see recipe page 194)

• Minced Beef Steaks (see recipe page 191 but increase beef mince to 400g) served with 200g fresh vegetables of your choice (excluding potatoes)

(P) ● Steak and Kidney Pie (see recipe page 195, but exclude potatoes) served with 250g boiled green vegetables. Plus 1 low-fat yogurt (max. 100 kcal and 5% fat)

● Beef and Beer Stew (recipe page 197) served with 250g green vegetables and carrots. Plus 1 piece fresh fruit

● Apple-Stuffed Pork Fillet (see recipe page 206) served with 300g boiled vegetables (excluding potatoes). Plus 1 blue Portion Pot® 2% fat Greek yogurt mixed with 1 red Portion Pot® (115g) raspberries

● 200g lean lamb steak, grilled, served with 250g vegetables (excluding potatoes) plus a little low-fat gravy and mint sauce

● Braised Lamb Shanks (see recipe page 200) served with unlimited fresh vegetables (excluding potatoes)

High-protein dinners: chicken and turkey

(approx. 400 kcal each)

(P) ● Quick and easy chicken curry: Dry-fry 1 × 150g chopped chicken breast (no skin) in a preheated non-stick pan with ½ chopped onion and 1 crushed garlic clove. Sprinkle 1 tsp curry powder over and 'cook out' for 1 minute, then add 1 small chopped chilli, ½ chopped green pepper, 25g button mushrooms (optional) and 400g tinned chopped tomatoes, and simmer for 5 minutes to reduce. Serve with 300g stir-fry vegetables plus 2 dsp raita (0% fat Greek yogurt mixed with a little mint sauce)

● 150g chicken breast (no skin) dry-fried with 100g sliced mushrooms then topped with ½ × 295g tin

Campbell's Condensed Low Fat Mushroom Soup and served with 200g boiled carrots and green vegetables

● Spicy Baked Chicken with Parsnips (see recipe page 222) served with 300g fresh vegetables (excluding potatoes). Plus 1 piece fresh fruit

● Oven-Baked Chicken Tikka Masala (see recipe page 219) served with a large mixed salad tossed in oil-free dressing

● Turkey stir-fry with ginger (serves 1): Chop 100g turkey breast (no skin) into bite-sized pieces and dry-fry in a non-stick pan with ½ crushed garlic clove. When the turkey has changed colour and is almost cooked through, add 1 chopped red or green pepper, 1 chopped celery stick, ½ chopped red onion, 25g mushrooms and 50g mangetout and dry-fry quickly but do not overcook. Just before serving add 1 tsp grated fresh ginger, soy sauce to taste and 2 tbsp roughly chopped fresh coriander and heat through for 30 seconds

● 4 turkey rashers and 1 low-fat pork sausage, grilled, served with 1 dry-fried egg, 1 yellow Portion Pot® (115g) baked beans, unlimited grilled mushrooms plus 400g tinned tomatoes boiled well to reduce

● Roast Turkey Leg Fricassee (see recipe page 229) served with 200g fresh vegetables of your choice (excluding potatoes)

High-protein dinners: fish (approx. 400 kcal each)

● 100g salmon steak, grilled, steamed or microwaved, served with 350g (1 bag) stir-fry vegetables, dry-fried, and a little reduced-salt soy sauce

- 200g white fish steamed, grilled or baked, served with 300g vegetables of your choice (excluding potatoes) plus ¼ pack Colman's Parsley Sauce mix made with semi-skimmed milk (in addition to allowance)
- 115g fresh salmon, steamed, grilled or microwaved, served with 1 yellow Portion Pot® (70g) frozen peas, 200g additional green vegetables and 1 dsp extra-light mayonnaise
- Red Pepper Houmous Baked Cod (see recipe page 248) served with unlimited fresh vegetables (excluding potatoes). Plus 1 low-fat yogurt (max. 100 kcal and 5% fat)
- Chinese Salmon Steaks with Stir-Fried Vegetables (see recipe page 235)

Dinners with dessert

Carbohydrate dinners with dessert: meat and chicken
(approx. 400 kcal each)

2 low-fat beef or pork sausages (max. 5% fat), grilled, served with 1 yellow Portion Pot® (100g) mashed sweet potato, plus 100g each spring greens or cabbage, 100g cauliflower or broccoli and a little low-fat gravy. Plus 1 low-sugar jelly, e.g. Hartley's (max. 10 kcal) served with 1 × 100ml scoop low-fat (max. 5% fat) ice cream (e.g. Wall's Soft Scoop) or other low-fat pudding (max. 75 kcal and 5% fat)

Chicken Korma (see recipe page 214) served with 30g (dry weight) boiled basmati rice. Plus 1 low-fat yogurt or other low-fat dessert (max. 100 kcal and 5% fat)

Ⓓ Ⓒ Any low-fat stir-fry ready meal, e.g. beef stir-fry or similar (max. 350 kcal and 5% fat) served with 150g beansprouts or mangetout. Plus 1 Hartley's Low Sugar Jelly (max. 10 kcal) and 120g fresh fruit salad, or other low-fat dessert of your choice (max. 70 kcal and 5% fat)

Ⓒ 100g lean roast chicken (no skin) served with 100g each dry-roast sweet potatoes, carrots and broccoli and a little low-fat gravy. Plus 1 meringue basket filled with 1 tsp 2% fat Greek yogurt and 50g strawberries

Ⓒ Jerk Chicken and Potato Bake (see recipe page 226) served with unlimited vegetables (excluding potatoes). Plus 150g fresh fruit salad

Ⓒ Turkey Spaghetti (see recipe page 228). Plus 100ml Ben & Jerry's frozen yogurt (any flavour) or any other low-fat dessert (max. 150 kcal and 5% fat)

Carbohydrate dinners with dessert: fish

(approx. 400 kcal each)

Ⓓ Ⓒ 100g white fish, steamed, grilled or baked, served with 115g new potatoes (boiled in skins), 200g additional green vegetables, plus ¼ pack Colman's Parsley Sauce mix (made up with milk from allowance). Plus 1 scoop Wall's Soft Scoop Light Ice Cream topped with 100g sliced strawberries or any other low-fat dessert of your choice (max. 90 kcal and 5% fat)

Ⓒ Seared Tuna with Chilli Cream (see recipe page 245) served with 150g dry-roasted potatoes and unlimited vegetables or salad. Plus 1 low-fat yogurt (max. 5% fat and 75 kcal)

D Ⓒ Sardine Tagliatelle (see recipe page 234) served with salad. Plus 1 low-fat ice cream or ice lolly (max. 100 kcal and 5% fat)

Ⓒ 125g smoked trout fillets served with a large mixed salad tossed in oil-free dressing. Plus 1 Ambrosia Crumble Pud (any flavour) or other low-fat dessert (max. 185 kcal and 5% fat)

Carbohydrate dinners with dessert: vegetarian

(approx. 400 kcal each)

D Ⓥ Ⓒ 1 green hole Portion Pot® (52g dry weight) spaghetti, boiled with a vegetable stock cube, served with ½ pot (175g) fresh tomato-based pasta sauce (max. 5% fat) topped with 20g grated low-fat mature cheese (max. 5% fat). Plus 1 low-fat yogurt or fromage frais (max. 100 kcal and 5% fat)

Ⓥ Ⓒ 1 Quorn Cottage Pie served with 100g each dry-roast sweet potatoes, carrots and broccoli and a little low-fat gravy. Plus 1 meringue basket filled with 1 tsp Total 2% Greek yogurt and 50g strawberries

Ⓥ Ⓒ Garlic Mushroom Spelt Spaghetti (see recipe page 259) served with a large salad. Plus 100g fresh fruit salad

Ⓥ Ⓒ 2 Quorn sausages, grilled, served with 1 yellow Portion Pot® (100g) mashed sweet potato, plus 100g each spring greens or cabbage, 100g cauliflower or broccoli and a little low-fat gravy. Plus 1 low-sugar jelly, e.g. Hartley's (max. 10 kcal) served with 1 × 100ml scoop low-fat (max. 5% fat) ice cream (e.g. Wall's Soft Scoop) or other low-fat pudding (max. 75 kcal and 5% fat)

(D) ✓ © 1 Quorn Peppered Steak, grilled or dry-fried, served with 100g low-fat oven chips (max. 5% fat) plus 2 sliced tomatoes, grilled, 50g grilled mushrooms and a large mixed salad tossed in oil-free dressing. Plus 100g fresh fruit salad

✓ © Quorn Rendang Curry (see recipe page 270) served with 1 blue Portion Pot® (55g dry weight) boiled basmati rice. Plus 100g fresh strawberries or raspberries

✓ © Aubergine and Artichoke Gratin (see recipe page 251) served with 100g boiled new potatoes and a large salad. Plus 1 meringue basket topped with 50g strawberries or raspberries and 2 tsp 0% fat Greek yogurt

✓ © Baby Courgette Pasta (see recipe page 263) served with a large salad. Plus 1 low-fat yogurt (max. 100 kcal and 5% fat)

✓ © Mushroom Biryani (see recipe page 275) served with a large salad tossed in oil-free dressing. Plus 1 Müller Fruit Corner yogurt or other low-fat dessert (max. 200 kcal and 5% fat)

✓ © Sweet Potato and Fruit Curry (see recipe page 276) served with 1 low-fat mini naan bread. Plus 1 low-fat yogurt (max. 70 kcal and 5% fat)

✓ © Any low-fat vegetarian ready meal, e.g. cottage pie or similar (max. 300 kcal and 5% fat) served with 100g broccoli. Plus 1 Hartley's sugar-free jelly and 120g fresh fruit salad, or other low-fat dessert of your choice (max. 70 kcal and 5% fat)

✓ © 3-egg omelette, dry-fried, filled with 50g low-fat mature cheese (max. 5% fat) and served with a large mixed salad tossed in oil-free dressing

(D) **(V)** **(C)** Tomato Risotto with Roasted Vegetables (see recipe page 256). Plus 1 individual meringue basket filled with 1 dsp 2% fat Greek yogurt topped with 100g strawberries or raspberries

High-protein dinners with dessert: meat and chicken
(approx. 400 kcal each)

(D) **(P)** 120g rump steak, grilled, served with a large mixed salad tossed in oil-free dressing plus 2 tomatoes, halved and grilled. Plus 1 meringue basket topped with 1 blue Portion Pot® (80g) 0% fat Greek yogurt and 1 yellow Portion Pot® (70g) blueberries or 1 red Portion Pot® (115g) raspberries, or any other low-fat dessert of your choice (max. 125 kcal and 5% fat)

(P) Chilli Con Carne (see recipe page 196) served with a large salad tossed in oil-free dressing. Plus 1 × 123g pot Dole Fruit Jelly or other low-fat dessert (max. 100 kcal and 5% fat)

(P) 150g lean lamb steak, grilled, served with 200g vegetables (excluding potatoes) plus a little low-fat gravy and mint sauce. Plus 1 Müllerlight banana and custard yogurt or other low-fat dessert (max. 100 kcal and 5% fat)

(P) Barbecue Pork Slices (see recipe page 205) served with 1 blue Portion Pot® (75g) tomato salsa plus unlimited fresh vegetables (excluding potatoes) or a large mixed salad. Plus 100g fresh fruit salad

(P) Basil and Tomato Cheese Stuffed Chicken (see recipe page 213) served with a large mixed salad. Plus 1 meringue basket filled with 2 tsp 0% fat Greek yogurt and topped with 25g sliced strawberries

(D) **℗** 100g roast beef or lamb or 125g roast pork served with 200g vegetables of your choice (excluding potatoes) and a little gravy made without fat. Plus 1 × 25g slice fat-free Swiss roll served with 50g low-fat custard, or any other low-fat pudding (max. 130 kcal and 5% fat)

℗ 100g chicken tikka breast fillets served with a large mixed salad drizzled with raita (2 dsp low-fat natural yogurt mixed with a little mint sauce). Plus 1 low-fat dessert or any other dessert of your choice (max. 200 kcal and 5% fat)

℗ Honey and Mustard Chicken (see recipe page 220) served with a large mixed salad. Plus 100g fresh fruit salad topped with 1 tsp 2% fat Greek yogurt

High-protein dinners with dessert: fish

(approx. 400 kcal each)

(D) **℗** Salmon with Spiced Cucumber (see recipe page 236) served with a small side salad. Plus 1 × 100 kcal low-fat dessert

℗ 130g salmon steak, steamed, microwaved or grilled, served with 100g broccoli, 100g mangetout and 1 tsp Thai sweet chilli dipping sauce mixed with 1 dsp extra-light mayonnaise. Plus 100g sliced strawberries topped with 1 tsp 2% fat Greek yogurt

℗ 80g salmon steak, steamed, microwaved or grilled, served with 100g mangetout and 1 tsp Thai sweet chilli dipping sauce mixed with 1 dsp extra-light mayonnaise. Plus Eton Mess: 1 meringue basket, broken up, mixed with 1 tbsp 2% fat Greek yogurt and 10 fresh raspberries

(D) **(P)** 1 rainbow trout, grilled, poached or barbecued with black pepper and lemon juice, served with 1 yellow Portion Pot® (70g) frozen peas and 100g carrots. Plus ¼ pack serving Angel Delight (strawberry or butterscotch flavour) made up with semi-skimmed milk (in addition to daily allowance)

(P) Seared Tuna with Chilli Cream (see recipe page 245) served with 200g green vegetables. Plus 1 scoop Wall's Soft Scoop Light Ice Cream topped with 100g sliced strawberries

(P) Seared Tuna with Chilli Cream (see recipe page 245) served with unlimited vegetables (excluding potatoes) or salad. Plus 1 low-fat yogurt or dessert (max. 200 kcal and 5% fat)

Rosemary Conley Solo Slim® Dinners

Solo Slim® meat dinners (approx. 400 kcal each)

(S) • 1 pouch Solo Slim® Low-Fat Spicy Mixed Bean Soup plus 1 pouch Solo Slim® Low-Fat Beef Goulash served with 100g green vegetables

• 1 pouch Solo Slim® Low-Fat Beef Goulash served with unlimited boiled green vegetables. Plus 115g strawberries served on a meringue basket and topped with 1 tbsp low-fat yogurt or fromage frais, or other low-fat dessert (max. 150 kcal and 5% fat)

• 1 pouch Solo Slim® Low-Fat Beef Bolognese served with a green salad. Plus 1 sliced kiwi fruit served on a meringue basket and topped with 1 dsp low-fat yogurt or fromage frais, or any other low fat dessert (max. 100 kcal and 5% fat)

(S)

- 1 pouch Solo Slim® Low-Fat Spicy Carrot and Coriander Soup plus 1 pouch Solo Slim® Low-Fat Beef Bolognese served with a small green salad
- 1 pouch Solo Slim® Low-Fat Beef Goulash served with 100g new potatoes (boiled in skins), plus 100g broccoli and 100g carrots
- 1 pouch Solo Slim® Low-Fat Beef Bolognese plus a large mixed salad tossed in oil-free dressing. Plus 1 satsuma
- 1 pouch Solo Slim® Low-Fat Carrot and Coriander Soup plus 1 pouch Solo Slim® Low-Fat Beef Meatballs and Potato
- 1 pouch Solo Slim® Low-Fat Chilli and Rice served with a large mixed salad tossed in oil-free dressing and 1 mini pitta bread
- 1 pouch Solo Slim® Low-Fat Chilli and Rice. Plus 1 Ambrosia Jelly Pud (jelly with custard) or other low-fat dessert (max. 130 kcal and 5% fat)
- 1 pouch Solo Slim® Low-Fat Lamb Hotpot served with 200g vegetables (excluding potatoes). Plus 1 piece fresh fruit
- 1 pouch Solo Slim® Low-Fat Lamb Hotpot served with 100g green vegetables. Plus 1 Solo Slim® Nutrition Bar (any flavour)
- 1 pouch Solo Slim® Low-Fat Lentil Soup plus 1 pouch Solo Slim® Low-Fat Lamb Hotpot
- 1 pouch Solo Slim® Low-Fat Sausage Casserole plus 200g fresh vegetables (excluding potatoes)
- 1 pouch Solo Slim® Low-Fat Leek and Potato Soup plus 1 pouch Solo Slim® Low-Fat Pork Meatballs with Smokey Beans. Plus 1 kiwi fruit or satsuma

Solo Slim® chicken dinners (approx. 400 kcal each)

(S) • 1 pouch Solo Slim® Low-Fat Thai Chicken Curry plus either 200g stir-fried vegetables or 1 pouch Solo Slim® Low-Fat Mushroom Soup

• 1 pouch Solo Slim® Low-Fat Carrot and Coriander Soup plus 1 pouch Solo Slim® Low-Fat Chicken Korma

• 1 pouch Solo Slim® Low-Fat Chicken Hotpot served with 200g fresh vegetables (excluding potatoes). Plus 150g fresh fruit salad or 1 Solo Slim® Nutrition Bar (any flavour)

• 1 pouch Solo Slim® Low-Fat Chicken Korma plus 100g beansprouts and 1 mini pitta bread

• 1 pouch Solo Slim® Low-Fat Thai Chicken Curry. Plus 1 low-fat chocolate mousse or other low-fat dessert (max. 100 kcal and 5% fat)

• 1 pouch Solo Slim® Low-Fat Thai Chicken Curry served with a large mixed salad tossed in oil-free dressing and 1 mini pitta bread

• 100g cooked chicken tikka breast fillets served with 1 pouch Solo Slim® Low-Fat Spicy Vegetable and Lentil Dhal

• 1 pouch Solo Slim® Low-Fat Thai Chicken Curry plus either 200g stir-fried vegetables or 1 pouch Solo Slim® Low-Fat Mushroom Soup

Solo Slim® vegetarian dinners (approx. 400 kcal each)

(S) ✔ 1 pouch Solo Slim® Low-Fat Minestrone Soup plus 1 pouch Solo Slim® Low-Fat Vegetable and Lentil Dhal served with 1 dsp mango chutney

✔ 1 pouch Solo Slim® Low-Fat Moroccan Spiced Chickpea Tagine. Plus 1 piece fresh fruit

(S) ✅ 1 pouch Solo Slim® Low-Fat Leek and Potato Soup plus 1 pouch Solo Slim® Low-Fat Moroccan Spiced Chickpea Tagine

✅ 1 pouch Solo Slim® Low-Fat Tomato and Vegetable Pasta served with a large side salad. Plus 1 low-fat yogurt (max. 100 kcal and 5% fat)

✅ 1 pouch Solo Slim® Low-Fat Butternut Squash Soup plus 1 pouch Solo Slim® Low-Fat Three Bean Casserole served with a large mixed salad

✅ 1 pouch Solo Slim® Low-Fat Mushroom Soup plus 1 pouch Solo Slim® Low-Fat Moroccan Spiced Chickpea Tagine served with a small salad tossed in oil-free dressing

✅ 1 pouch Solo Slim® Low-Fat Chunky Vegetable Soup plus 1 pouch Solo Slim® Low-Fat Mushroom Stroganoff served with 200g boiled green vegetables

Dinner recipes using Rosemary Conley cooking sauces
(approx. 400 kcal each)

Rosemary Conley Low-Fat Tomato and Basil Sauce:

(C) ● Pancetta Risotto with Tomato and Basil Sauce (see recipe page 210)

● Sausage Penne with Tomato and Basil Sauce (see recipe page 212). Plus 1 low-fat yogurt (max. 100 kcal and 5% fat)

Rosemary Conley Low-Fat Tomato and Chilli Sauce:

(C) ● Arrabbiata Prawns (see recipe page 241) served with 1 red Portion Pot® (80g dry weight) pasta shapes

Spicy Tagliatelle with Tomato and Chilli Sauce (see recipe page 280) served with a large mixed salad tossed in oil-free dressing. Plus 1 pot low-fat yogurt (max 100 kcal and 5% fat)

Rosemary Conley Low-Fat Thai Red Sauce:

● Red Thai Chicken Curry (see recipe page 227) served with 40g (dry weight) boiled basmati rice

Rosemary Conley Low-Fat Tikka Masala Sauce:

● Chicken Tikka Masala (see recipe page 215) served with 40g (dry weight) boiled basmati rice
● Tikka Salmon (see recipe page 240) plus 1 mini pitta bread

Rosemary Conley Low-Fat Jerk Barbecue Sauce:

● Jerk Barbecue Pork and Prune Kebabs (see recipe page 208) served with a large mixed salad tossed in oil-free dressing
● Easy Jerk Barbecue Chicken (see recipe page 223) served with a large mixed salad tossed in oil-free dressing

Rosemary Conley Low-Fat Piri Piri Sauce:

● Piri Piri Pork (see recipe page 209) served with 40g (dry weight) boiled basmati rice

Power Snacks

All the following snacks are approx. 50 kcal each. Choose two Power Snacks a day (or more if your calorie allowance permits). You can eat your Power Snacks at any time of day, but eating one mid-morning and one mid-afternoon will help stave off hunger pangs between meals.

Fruit and yogurt (approx. 50 kcal each)
- 1 small apple or pear
- 1 nectarine or peach
- 1 medium orange
- 1 fun-size mini banana
- 90g blueberries
- 100g cherries
- 1 kiwi fruit plus 6 grapes
- 12 seedless grapes
- ½ fresh mango (approx. 80g)
- 50g sliced mango with 100g chopped melon
- 150g sliced fresh strawberries
- 50g sliced mango mixed with 75g sliced fresh strawberries
- 200g rhubarb, stewed, sweetened with low-calorie sweetener and served with 1 dsp low-fat yogurt
- 150g fresh fruit salad
- 200g fresh melon
- 100g fresh melon plus 1 red Portion Pot® (115g) raspberries
- 1 peach with 1 dsp low-fat yogurt
- 100g fresh pineapple
- 2 satsumas
- 1 yellow Portion Pot® (70g) blueberries served with 1 tsp 2% fat Greek yogurt

- 1 red Portion Pot® (115g) raspberries topped with 1 tsp 2% fat Greek yogurt
- 1 blue Portion Pot® (80g) low-fat fromage frais
- ½ fresh grapefruit sprinkled with 1 tsp sugar
- 1 Hartley's Low Sugar jelly (max. 10 kcal) plus 1 yellow Portion Pot® (70g) blueberries
- 1 Hartley's Low Sugar Jelly (max. 10 kcal) plus 1 kiwi or passion fruit
- 1 low-fat yogurt (max. 50 kcal and 5% fat)
- 3 dried apricots
- 15g raisins or sultanas

Other Power Snacks (approx. 50 kcal each)
- 1 Ryvita spread with Marmite and topped with 1 dsp low-fat cottage cheese
- 1 brown Ryvita or rice cake spread with 20g extra-light soft cheese (max 5% fat) and topped with fresh basil leaves and 2 cherry tomatoes
- ½ Solo Slim® Nutrition Bar (any flavour)
- 1 blue Portion Pot® (15g) Special K cereal eaten dry like crisps or served with milk from allowance
- 1 cereal bowlful of salad
- Carrot and sultana salad: 100g grated carrot mixed with 10 sultanas and tossed in oil-free dressing
- Vegetable nibble box: 80g carrot, 60g cucumber and 2 sticks celery cut into crudités plus 2 cherry tomatoes
- 12 cherry tomatoes
- 10 cherry tomatoes sprinkled with basil and a little balsamic vinegar
- 20g low-fat mature cheese (max. 5% fat) plus 2 cherry tomatoes and 1 celery stick
- 40g cooked, shelled prawns mixed with shredded lettuce leaves and a little oil-free salad dressing

- 40g chicken tikka mini fillets served with shredded lettuce leaves
- 20g wafer-thin ham plus 1 sliced tomato, 2 slices cucumber and a few salad leaves
- 1 grilled turkey rasher plus 1 grilled large tomato
- 1 beef tomato sprinkled with basil plus 2 spring onions

Treats and Desserts

If your calorie allowance permits, choose a high-fat treat *or* an alcoholic drink (max. 100 kcal) each day *plus* a low-fat treat or dessert (max. 100 kcal). Alternatively, you can save up your treats and alcohol calories over seven days for a special occasion or treat.

High-Fat Treats

Chocolate (100 kcal or less)
- 1 Aero Biscuit 99 kcal 29.4% fat
- 4 Rolos 98 kcal 20.3% fat
- 21.9g Milky Way 98 kcal 16.1% fat
- Jaffa Cakes cake bar 96 kcal 14.2% fat
- Cadbury Dairy Milk Freddo Caramel 95 kcal 24.5% fat
- McVitie's Penguin Wafer 94 kcal 30.1% fat
- 2 Nestlé Celebrations 92 kcal 27.1% fat
- 2 Jaffa Cakes 92 kcal 8% fat
- 3 Cadbury Fingers 90 kcal 27% fat
- Fun Size Chocolate Cupcake 89 kcal 25.3% fat
- 15g bar Green & Black's Organic Chocolate 84 kcal 35.3% fat
- 1 McVitie's Milk Chocolate Digestive 84 kcal 23.4% fat

Crisps and savoury snacks (100 kcal or less)
- 2 Quorn Mini Savoury Eggs 100 kcal 11.5% fat
- 21g bag Wotsits 99 kcal 33% fat
- 25g bag Walkers Baked Ready Salted 98 kcal 8% fat
- 25g bag Jacob's Twiglets 97 kcal 11.9% fat
- Jacob's Snack Pack – Choice Grain 93 kcal 13.9% fat
- 4 Bassett's Liquorice Allsorts 91 kcal 4.9% fat

- 22g bag Snack a Jacks Salt & Vinegar 89 kcal 7.4% fat
- 16.4g bag Quavers 87 kcal 30% fat
- 20g Velvet Crunch Sweet Potato Snacks 80 kcal 9.8% fat
- 2 × 10g mini Peperami 76 kcal 30% fat
- 1 Dairylea Strip Cheese 73 kcal 27.5% fat

Sweet treats (100 kcal or less)
- 11 Mikado biscuits 99 kcal 19% fat
- Kellogg's Special K Mini Breaks Chocolate 99 kcal 10% fat
- 6 Starburst Twisted Chews 99 kcal 7.3% fat
- Harvest Chewee Milk Choc Chip 92 kcal 14.5% fat
- Go Ahead Fruity Cake Slice (Honey, Caramel & Sultana) 89 kcal 7.6% fat
- Kellogg's Rice Krispies Snack Bar 83 kcal 11% fat
- Golden Syrup Pancakes 80 kcal 5.7% fat
- Ryvita Fruit Crunch 54 kcal 5.4% fat
- Chocolate Whoopie Cakes (see recipe page 292) 88 kcal 7.6% fat
- Flapjack (see recipe page 293) 84 kcal 7% fat

Low-fat Treats and Desserts

Desserts (200 kcal or less)
- Blueberry and Lemon Muffins (see recipe page 287) 198 kcal 4.3% fat
- Macaroons (see recipe page 288) 138 kcal 0.6% fat
- Ramekin Cheesecakes (see recipe page 290) 134 kcal 4.7% fat
- Raspberry Traybake (see recipe page 289) 121 kcal 4.2% fat

- Lemon and Blueberry Pancakes (see recipe page 284) 115 kcal 3.8% fat
- Blueberry Chocolate Soufflés (see recipe page 281) 106 kcal 1.6% fat
- Chocolate Frozen Yogurt (see recipe page 282) 81 kcal 0.6% fat

Sweet treats/desserts (100 kcal or less)
- 1 bag Iced Gems 99 kcal 3.1% fat
- Solero Berry Berry Lolly 99 kcal 1.5% fat
- The Skinny Cow Caramel Shortcake Lolly 93 kcal 2.9% fat
- Special K Red Berry Bar 88 kcal 5% fat
- 180ml pouch Innocent Fruit Smoothie Strawberries, Blackberries & Raspberries 81 kcal 0% fat
- 50g pot Müller Little Stars Fromage Frais 53 kcal 4% fat
- 1 Snack a Jacks Caramel 51 kcal 2.1% fat

Savoury treats (100 kcal or less)
- 24g bag (from multipack) Ryvita Minis Salt & Vinegar 75 kcal 2.8% fat
- 2 × Snack a Jacks Cheese Flavour 76 kcal 2.5% fat
- Whitworths Bite Size Apricots 35g Snack Pack 70 kcal 0.3% fat
- The Fruit Factory Fruit String (20g bag) 64 kcal 0.4% fat
- Alpen Light Summer Fruits 61 kcal 4% fat
- Whitworths Bite Size Prunes 35g Snack Pack 60 kcal 0.4% fat

Alcoholic Drinks

Use slimline mixers and diet drinks with spirits to keep the calories down.

Beer
bitter 300ml (½ pint) 91 kcal
lager 300ml (½ pint) 82 kcal

Brandy and liqueurs
25ml measure brandy 50 kcal
25ml measure Southern Comfort 81 kcal
25ml measure Tia Maria 75 kcal

Spirits (use low-cal mixers)
25ml measure Bacardi 56 kcal
275ml bottle Diet Bacardi Breezer 96 kcal
25ml measure gin 50 kcal
25ml measure vodka 50 kcal
25ml measure whisky 50 kcal

Vermouth
50ml measure Martini Rosso 70 kcal
50ml measure Martini Extra Dry 48 kcal

Wine and fortified wine
1 yellow Portion Pot (125ml glass) Champagne 95 kcal
1 yellow Portion Pot (125ml glass) dry white wine 83 kcal
1 yellow Portion Pot (125ml glass) medium white wine 93 kcal
1 yellow Portion Pot (125ml glass) red wine 85 kcal
1 yellow Portion Pot (125ml glass) medium rosé wine 89 kcal
50ml measure port 79 kcal
50ml measure sweet sherry 68 kcal
50ml measure dry sherry 58 kcal

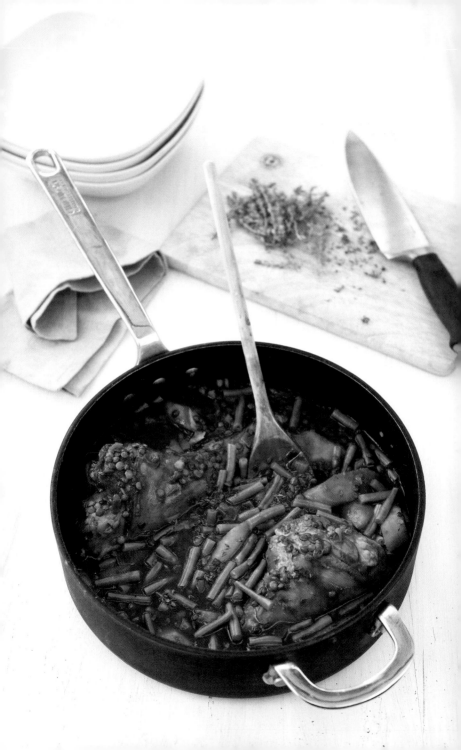

9
Recipes

Note: All calorie and fat figures per serving exclude any accompaniments not listed in the ingredients.

Braised Lamb Shanks (see recipe on page 200).

Soups

Cauliflower and Spinach Soup ⓥ

Per serving 96 calories 1% fat
Serves 4 Prep time 5 mins Cook time 20 mins

1 large onion, diced
1 small cauliflower (about 600g), broken into florets
2 garlic cloves, crushed
1 tsp ground coriander
2 tsp vegetable stock powder
200g fresh leaf spinach
salt and freshly ground black pepper, to taste
2% fat Greek yogurt, to serve

1 Put the onion, cauliflower, garlic, coriander and
   vegetable stock powder in a large saucepan and cover
   with water. Bring to the boil and simmer gently until the
   cauliflower is soft and cooked.
2 Allow the soup to cool slightly, then pour into a liquidiser
   and blend until smooth, adding the fresh spinach in
   batches. Return the soup to the saucepan to reheat,
   adding more seasoning and adjusting the consistency by
   adding boiling water if required.
3 Pour the soup into warmed serving bowls and add a swirl
   of yogurt to each bowl.

Chilli Bean Soup ✓

Per serving 163 calories 1% fat
Serves 4 Prep time 5 mins Cook time 25 mins

1 red onion, finely chopped
1 small red chilli, sliced
200g tin chickpeas, drained and rinscd
200g tin red kidney beans, drained and rinsed
400g tin chopped tomatoes
600ml (1 pint) vegetable stock
1 tbsp tomato purée
2 tsp chopped fresh oregano
salt and freshly ground black pepper, to taste

1 Heat a non-stick wok or frying pan and dry-fry the red
   onion and chilli for 4–5 minutes.
2 Transfer to a large saucepan, add the remaining
   ingredients and simmer gently for 20 minutes. Season to
   taste with salt and pepper before serving.

Sweet Potato and Leek Soup ✓

Per serving 122 calories 1% fat
Serves 4 Prep time 10 mins Cook time 40 mins

2 large leeks, chopped
300g sweet potato, peeled and diced
2 garlic cloves, crushed
1 litre vegetable stock
300ml (½ pint) semi-skimmed milk
fresh chives, to garnish

1 Heat a large non-stick saucepan and dry-fry the leeks for
   1–2 minutes until soft. Add the potatoes, garlic and stock
   and bring to a gentle simmer. Cook for about 35–40
   minutes, or until the potato is soft.
2 Pour in the milk and bring back up to near boiling.
   Sprinkle with chives and serve.

Roasted Aubergine, Pepper and Chilli Soup ⓥ

Per serving 79 calories 0.4% fat
Serves 4 Prep time 10 mins Cook time 30 mins

1 large aubergine
2 garlic cloves, chopped
2 red onions, chopped
500ml vegetable stock
400g tin chopped tomatoes
1 red pepper, deseeded and diced
1 small red chilli, sliced

1 Preheat the oven to 200°C, 400°F, Gas Mark 6. Chop the aubergine into chunky dice and place in a roasting tin with the chopped garlic. Roast, uncovered, in the oven for 10 minutes or until soft. You can roast for longer if you prefer a stronger flavour.
2 Transfer the aubergine to a saucepan, add the remaining ingredients and simmer gently for 20 minutes, or until the vegetables are cooked.

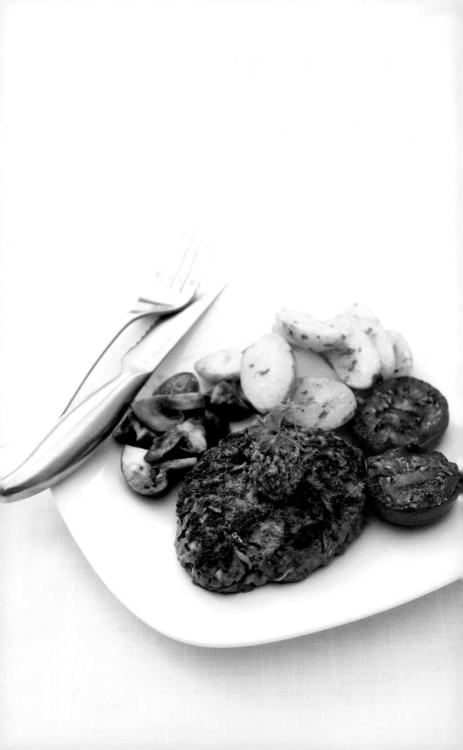

Beef and Lamb

Minced Beef Steaks

Per serving 182 calories 4.6% fat
Serves 4 Prep time 5 mins (plus chilling time)
Cook time 20 mins

300g extra-lean minced beef
100g Quorn mince
2 garlic cloves, crushed
1 red onion, finely chopped
1 courgette, grated
1 tsp grain mustard or horseradish sauce
1 tsp vegetable stock powder
salt and freshly ground black pepper, to taste

1 Combine all the ingredients in a bowl and season with salt and black pepper. Divide the mixture into 4 portions and, using your hands, mould each portion into a ball. Place on a board and use a palette knife to shape each ball into a teardrop shape. Chill in the fridge for 10 minutes.
2 Heat a non-stick griddle pan and dry-fry the steaks for 10 minutes on each side.

Ginger Beef Stir-Fry with Noodles

Per serving 338 calories 1.5% fat
Serves 4 Prep time 5 mins Cook time 10 mins

450g lean rump steak cut into strips
3 baby leeks, finely sliced
100g chestnut mushrooms, sliced
1 tbsp light soy sauce
1 tbsp sweet chilli sauce
1 tsp chopped fresh ginger
150g sugar snap peas, halved
2 whole pak choi
300g pack beansprouts
400g pack ready-to-wok medium noodles
1 tbsp chopped fresh coriander, to garnish

1 Heat a non-stick wok or frying pan and dry-fry the beef strips for 3–4 minutes until sealed. Remove from the pan and set aside on a plate.
2 Return the pan to the heat, add the leeks and mushrooms and dry-fry for 2–3 minutes, mixing well.
3 In a bowl or jug, mix together the soy and chilli sauces and the chopped ginger and pour over the beef, coating the meat.
4 Return the beef to the pan. Add the remaining ingredients, toss well to combine and then continue cooking until the meat is hot. Serve straight away garnished with the chopped coriander.

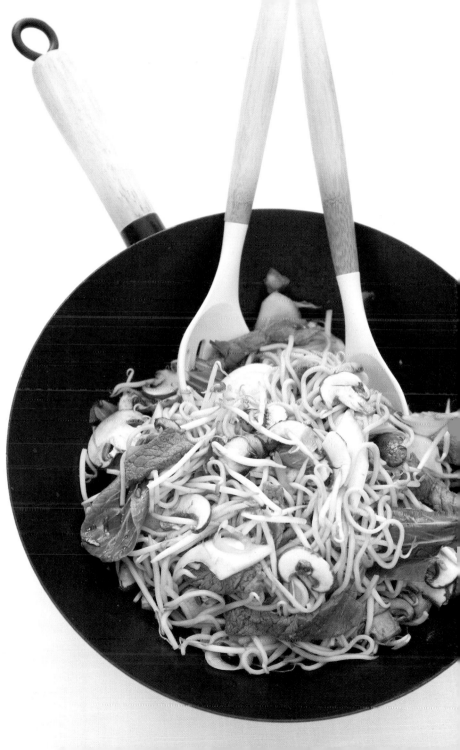

Oriental Beef Stir-Fry

Per serving 417 calories 1.2% fat
Serves 4 Prep time 5 mins (plus 10 mins marinating)
Cook time 10–15 mins

1 tbsp teriyaki sauce
1 tbsp light soy sauce
350g lean beef steak, cut into strips
3 baby leeks, finely sliced
2 carrots, finely shredded
100g chestnut mushrooms, sliced
150g sugar snap peas, cut in half
300g pack beansprouts
2 whole pak choi, chopped
100g tenderstem broccoli
100g baby corn
1 tbsp chopped fresh coriander, to serve

1 Mix together the teriyaki and soy sauce in a large bowl, add the beef and allow to marinate for 10 minutes.
2 Heat a non-stick wok or frying pan and stir-fry the beef strips for 3–4 minutes until sealed. Remove from the pan and set to one side.
3 Return the pan to the heat, add the leeks, carrots and mushrooms and stir–fry for 2–3 minutes, mixing well. Add the remaining vegetables and return the beef to the pan for 3–4 minutes.
4 Transfer to serving plates and sprinkle with fresh coriander.

Steak and Kidney Pie

Per serving 365 calories 1.3% fat
Serves 4 Prep time 25 mins Cook time 30–40 mins

200g lean rump or
  sirloin steak
200g kidneys, cut into
  bite-sized pieces
2 medium onions, chopped
300ml (½ pint) water
125ml red wine

2 beef stock cubes
1 tbsp gravy powder
900g potatoes, peeled
2 tbsp low-fat natural yogurt
4–5 tbsp skimmed milk
salt and freshly ground
  black pepper, to taste

1 Preheat the oven to 180°C, 350°F, Gas Mark 4, and
  preheat a large non-stick frying pan. Trim the steak,
  removing all visible fat, then cut the steak into cubes.
2 Dry-fry the cubes of beef steak and kidneys in the hot
  pan until well browned. Transfer the meat to a 30 x 20cm
  pie dish.
3 Add the onions to the pan and dry-fry until soft. Add the
  onions to the meat in the pie dish, pour the water and wine
  into the pan, add the stock cubes and bring to the boil.
4 Mix the gravy powder with a little cold water and add to
  the boiling stock in the pan, stirring continuously. The
  gravy should be quite thick, so add more gravy powder if
  necessary. Pour the gravy over the meat in the pie dish.
5 Boil the potatoes, then drain them and mash them with
  the yogurt and sufficient skimmed milk to make the
  consistency quite soft. Season to taste.
6 Carefully spoon the 'creamed' potato on top of the meat
  and gravy, covering it completely, then spread it carefully
  with a fork. Bake in the oven for 30–40 minutes, or until
  crisp and brown on top.

Chilli Con Carne

Per serving 246 calories 2.5% fat
Serves 6 Prep time 10 mins Cook time 25 mins

1 large onion, diced
2 garlic cloves, crushed
450g extra-lean minced beef
1 tbsp chopped fresh thyme
1 beef stock cube
1 red pepper, deseeded and thinly sliced
1 small red chilli, sliced
400g tin chopped tomatoes
400g tin kidney beans
300ml (½ pint) tomato passata
1 tbsp tomato purée
salt and freshly ground black pepper, to taste
chopped fresh parsley, to garnish

1 Heat a non-stick pan, and dry-fry the onion and garlic
   until soft. Add the mince and thyme, and continue
   cooking to brown the mince.
2 Sprinkle the stock cube over the mince, then add the red
   pepper, chilli, tomatoes, kidney beans, tomato passata
   and tomato purée. Simmer gently for 25 minutes until
   the sauce has thickened and the beef is tender. Serve
   garnished with fresh parsley.

Beef and Beer Stew

Per serving 256 calories 2.2% fat
Serves 4 Prep time 10 mins Cook time 1 hr

2 red onions, diced
2 garlic cloves, crushed
400g lean diced beef
2 celery sticks, chopped
10g sundried tomatoes, chopped
500ml beer or stout
500ml beef stock
1 tbsp low-fat gravy granules
250g small button mushrooms
1 tbsp mixed herbs (e.g. parsley, thyme, chives)
salt and freshly ground black pepper, to taste

1 Heat a large non-stick frying pan or wok and dry-fry the
   onions and garlic until they start to brown. Add the diced
   beef, season with salt and black pepper and continue
   cooking to seal the meat.
2 Add the celery, tomatoes and the beer or stout and bring
   to the boil. Stir in the beef stock and gravy granules, add
   the mushrooms and herbs, then cover with a lid and
   simmer gently for 1 hour until the meat is tender.
3 When the meat is tender, adjust the consistency of the
   sauce by adding more gravy granules or water and serve
   straight away.

Spicy Mexican Beef

Per serving 192 calories 1.6% fat
Serves 4 Prep time 10 mins Cook time 20 mins

400g rump steak, sliced
1 medium onion, diced
2 garlic cloves, crushed
1 green pepper, deseeded and diced
200g chestnut mushrooms, sliced
2 tsp fajita spice mix
1 tbsp chopped fresh mixed herbs
    (e.g. oregano, chives, parsley)
1 tbsp reduced-salt soy sauce
200g cherry tomatoes
100g cooked new potatoes, sliced
chilli sauce, for drizzling

1 Preheat a non-stick frying pan. Remove all visible fat
    from the beef. Add the onion, garlic and green pepper to
    the hot pan and dry-fry until soft.
2 Add the beef slices and lightly seal, then stir in the
    mushrooms, spice mix, herbs and soy sauce. Toss well
    together, then add the cherry tomatoes and sliced
    potatoes and heat through. Just before serving, drizzle
    with the chilli sauce.

Top right: Spicy Mexican Beef
Right: Braised Lamb Shanks (see recipe page 200)

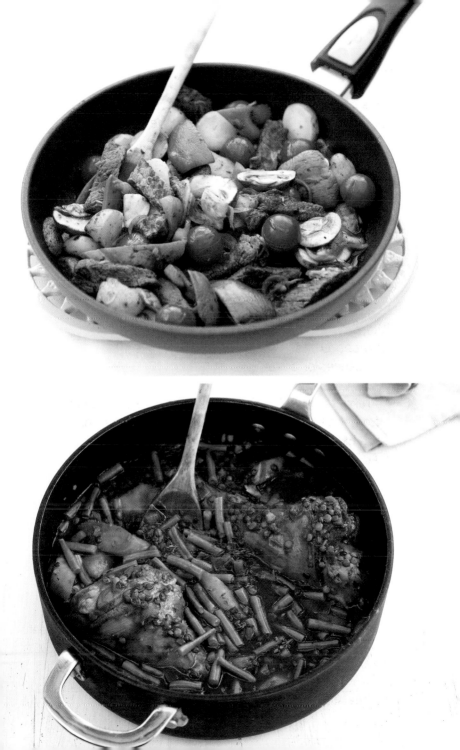

Braised Lamb Shanks

Per serving 253 calories 2.2% fat
Serves 4 Prep time 10 mins Cook time 1 hr 20 mins

500g lamb shanks, all visible fat removed
1 medium red onion, finely chopped
2 garlic cloves, crushed
4 parsnips, peeled and chopped
300g button mushrooms
1 tbsp tomato purée
500ml vegetable stock
2 tbsp green lentils
1 tbsp chopped mixed herbs
2 tsp gravy powder
200g fine green beans, chopped
salt and freshly ground black pepper, to taste
2 tbsp chopped fresh parsley, to serve

1 Preheat a large non-stick frying pan. Trim any traces of fat from the lamb and season with salt and black pepper.
2 Cook the shanks in the hot pan to seal them on all sides, then add the onion, garlic, parsnips and mushrooms and cook quickly over a high heat to soften the onion. Add the tomato purée, vegetable stock, lentils and herbs, stirring well. Dilute the gravy powder with a little cold water and stir into the pan, then cover and simmer for 1 hour to allow the lamb to cook through.
3 When the meat is tender, stir in the green beans, topping up with more stock if required, and cook for a further 20 minutes. Just before serving, stir in the fresh parsley. Serve straight away.

Illustrated on page 199 (bottom)

Mint Salsa Lamb Steak

Per serving 166 calories 3.9% fat
Serves 4 Prep time 10 mins (plus 30 mins marinating)
Cook time 20 mins

4 lean lamb leg steaks
4 tbsp dry sherry
2 garlic cloves, crushed
4–5 sprigs fresh rosemary
salt and freshly ground black pepper, to taste

for the salsa
1 green pepper, deseeded and diced
1 small green chilli, chopped
4 spring onions, chopped
1 tbsp chopped fresh mint
2 tbsp 2% fat Greek yogurt

1 Remove and discard all visible fat from the lamb steaks
   with a sharp knife. Place the steaks in a shallow
   container and season with salt and black pepper.
2 Combine the sherry, garlic and rosemary in a small bowl,
   mixing well. Pour over the lamb, then turn the steaks
   over to ensure both sides get coated. Leave to marinate
   for 30 minutes.
3 Mix together the salsa ingredients.
4 Heat a non-stick griddle pan, and cook the lamb steaks
   for 4–5 minutes on each side. Allow to rest for 2 minutes
   before serving with the salsa.

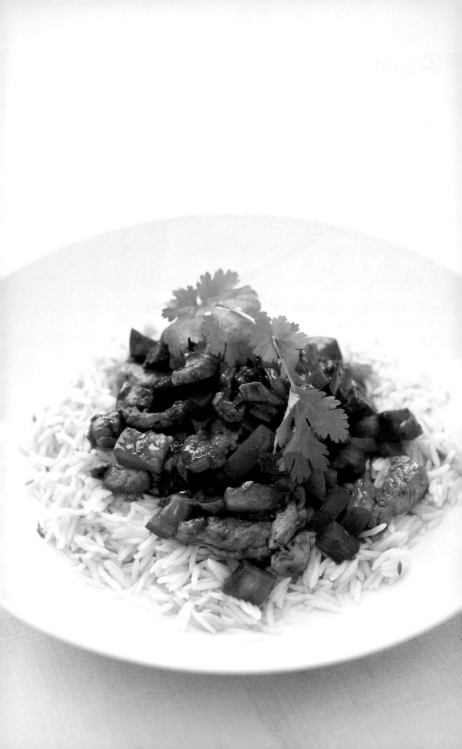

Pork

Black Bean Pork

Per serving 170 calories 1.6% fat
Serves 4 Prep time 10 mins Cook time 20 mins

1 red onion, chopped
2 garlic cloves, crushed
340g lean diced pork
1 aubergine, diced
2cm piece fresh ginger, peeled and finely chopped
1 tbsp low-salt soy sauce
120g black bean sauce
2 tomatoes, diced
salt and freshly ground black pepper, to taste
fresh coriander, to garnish

1 Heat a non-stick wok, and dry-fry the onion and garlic
   until soft. Add the diced pork and aubergine and
   continue cooking until the meat is sealed.
2 Stir in the remaining ingredients and mix well. Simmer
   gently for 10 minutes, or until the meat is tender and
   cooked through. Serve hot, garnished with coriander

Pork and Red Pepper Burgers

Per serving 144 calories 3.1% fat
Serves 4 Prep time 10 mins Cook time 10–15 mins

400g lean minced pork
1 red pepper, deseeded and finely diced
1 tsp vegetable stock powder
2 garlic cloves, crushed
1 tbsp chopped fresh mixed herbs
freshly ground black pepper, to taste

1 Preheat the grill to high.
2 Place all the ingredients together in a mixing bowl and
   season with black pepper. Divide the mixture into 4 and
   mould into burger shapes, squashing each one flat with
   your hands.
3 Cook the burgers under the hot grill for 10–15 minutes,
   turning them regularly. To test if they are cooked, insert a
   knife into the centre of one of the burgers; if the juices
   run clear and the flesh is not pink, they are ready.

Barbecue Pork Slices

Per serving 209 calories 2.9% fat
Serves 4 Prep time 10 mins (plus marinating time)
Cook time 15–20 mins

500g piece pork fillet
salt and freshly ground black pepper, to taste

for the marinade
pinch of cumin seeds
2 tbsp sweet chilli sauce
2 tbsp runny honey
1 tbsp Worcestershire sauce
2 garlic cloves, chopped
150ml (¼ pint) tomato passata

1 Remove all visible fat from the pork. Slice the pork into
   strips and season with salt and black pepper, then place
   in the bottom of an ovenproof dish.
2 Combine the marinade ingredients in a mixing bowl and
   pour over the pork. Leave to marinate for at least 1 hour.
3 Heat a health grill or barbecue, then cook the pork for
   15–20 minutes, turning it halfway through, until cooked
   through to the centre. Serve straight from the grill.

Apple-Stuffed Pork Fillet

Per serving 217 calories 3% fat
Serves 4 Prep time 15 mins Cook time 30 mins

450g lean pork fillet
2 eating apples, cored and diced
120g Quark low-fat soft cheese
1 tbsp chopped fresh sage
1 garlic clove, crushed
2 slices (50g) Parma ham
salt and freshly ground black pepper, to taste

1 Preheat the oven to 200°C, 400°F, Gas Mark 6.
2 Remove all visible fat from the pork and place the pork
   on a chopping board. Using a sharp knife, cut the fillet
   down the centre but not all the way through. Open up the
   pork into a flat piece of meat.
3 Mix together the apple, Quark, sage and garlic and
   season with salt and black pepper. Spread the mixture
   over the pork, then roll up the pork and wrap the Parma
   ham around the fillet and place in a non-stick roasting tin.
4 Roast in the oven for 30 minutes until cooked.

Pork and Leek Casserole

Per serving 242 calories 2% fat
Serves 2 Prep time 10 mins Cook time 30 mins

1 leek, trimmed and chopped
1 garlic clove, chopped
200g diced pork
1 tbsp Madeira wine
295g tin condensed low-fat mushroom soup
100ml rice milk

1 Heat a large non-stick pan and dry-fry the leek and garlic
   until soft. Add the pork and continue cooking until the
   meat is sealed. Stir in the Madeira
   wine, then the soup and simmer
   gently for 15 minutes.
2 Just before serving stir
   in the rice milk.

Jerk Barbecue Pork and Prune Kebabs

Per serving 337 calories 1.3% fat
Serves 2 Prep time 10 mins (plus marinating time)
Cook time 20 mins

200g pork fillet
1 red pepper, deseeded and diced
8 ready-to-eat prunes
200g pouch Rosemary Conley Low-Fat Jerk
    Barbecue Sauce
salt and freshly ground black pepper, to taste
1 tbsp chopped fresh mint, to garnish

1 Cut the pork into chunks. Take 2 wooden or metal
   skewers and thread alternate pieces of pork, peppers
   and prunes onto each skewer. Place on a non-stick
   baking tray, season with salt and black pepper, then
   drizzle with the jerk barbecue sauce. Leave to marinate
   for 30 minutes.
2 Preheat the grill to high (or preheat a barbecue). When
   ready to cook, grill the kebabs for 8–10 minutes on each
   side. Serve hot, garnished with chopped fresh mint.

Piri Piri Pork

Per serving 232 calories 2.5% fat
Serves 2 Prep time 10 mins Cook time 20 mins

2 × 100g pork steaks
200g pouch Rosemary Conley Low-Fat Piri Piri Sauce
1 tbsp runny honey
1 tbsp Worcestershire sauce
salt and freshly ground black pepper, to taste

1 Preheat a non-stick griddle pan. Remove any visible fat from the pork steaks, then season the steaks on both sides with salt and black pepper.
2 Add the steaks to the hot pan, browning them on both sides. Stir in the piri piri sauce, honey and Worcestershire sauce and continue to cook for 5 minutes.

Pancetta Risotto with Tomato and Basil Sauce

Per serving 339 calories 3.7% fat
Serves 2 Prep time 5 mins Cook time 35 mins

1 small red onion, finely chopped
1 garlic clove, crushed
50g pancetta, chopped
100g (dry weight) Arborio risotto rice
1 tbsp white wine
200g pouch Rosemary Conley Low-Fat Tomato
    and Basil Sauce
400ml vegetable stock
1 tbsp chopped fresh parsley
salt and freshly ground black pepper, to taste
a little low-fat mature cheese (max. 5% fat), to serve

1 Heat a large non-stick frying pan and dry-fry the onion
   and garlic until soft. Add the pancetta, rice and wine,
   add the sauce then gradually stir in the stock, allowing
   the rice to absorb it before adding more – this will take
   about 15–20 minutes.
2 Once all the liquid has been added, season with salt and
   black pepper to taste. Just before serving, stir in the
   parsley. Serve in warmed bowls and top with a little
   grated cheese.

Cheese, Bacon and Tomato Panini

Per serving 308 calories 4.3% fat
Serves 2 Prep time 5–10 mins

2 × 70g panini
3 tbsp extra-light mayonnaise
2 tbsp tomato ketchup
2 rashers lean back bacon, finely diced
6 cherry tomatoes, sliced
15g low-fat mature cheese (max. 5% fat), grated

1 Preheat the grill to high.
2 Split each panini in half, put on a non-stick baking tray,
   place under the grill and lightly toast on both sides.
3 Spread the mayo and ketchup on the panini. Sprinkle the
   remaining ingredients on top and return to the grill until
   the cheese has melted and the bacon cooked. Serve hot.

Sausage Penne with Tomato and Basil Sauce

Per serving 300 calories 1.8% fat
Serves 2 Prep time 20 mins Cook time 25 mins

2 low-fat pork sausages (max. 5% fat)
90g penne pasta
1 vegetable stock cube
1 red onion, sliced
1 garlic clove crushed
1 red pepper, deseeded and diced
200g pouch Rosemary Conley Low-Fat Tomato
   and Basil Sauce
salt and freshly ground black pepper, to taste
8 fresh basil leaves, to garnish

1 Grill the sausages until cooked and set aside. Cook the pasta in a pan of boiling water with the vegetable stock cube.
2 Meanwhile, heat a non-stick pan and dry-fry the onion, garlic and red pepper until soft. Stir in the tomato and basil sauce and simmer gently. Chop the cooked sausages into pieces and add to the sauce.
3 Drain the pasta and transfer to a serving dish. Pour the sauce over the pasta and sprinkle with fresh basil leaves.

Chicken and Turkey

Basil and Tomato Cheese Stuffed Chicken

Per serving 221 calories 1.1% fat
Serves 4 Prep time 10 mins Cook time 30–35 mins

4 skinless chicken breasts
4 thin slices (30g total) low-fat mature cheese
  (max. 5% fat)
8 fresh basil leaves
12 small cherry tomatoes
1 tsp ground coriander
1 tbsp thick balsamic vinegar
salt and freshly ground black pepper, to taste

1 Preheat the oven to 200°C, 400°F, Gas Mark 6.
2 Place the chicken breasts on a chopping board and slice
  each fillet open. Season with salt and black pepper, then
  place 1 slice of cheese, 2 basil leaves and 3 tomatoes in
  each fillet and fold back together. Place on a non-stick
  baking tray and dust the tops with ground coriander.
3 Bake in the oven for 30–35 minutes, depending on the
  thickness of the fillets. Transfer to serving plates, drizzle
  with balsamic vinegar and serve.

Chicken Korma

Per serving 233 calories 1.5% fat
Serves 4 Prep time 10 mins Cook time 20 mins

1 medium onion, chopped
2 garlic cloves, crushed
450g diced lean chicken
2 tbsp mild curry powder
1 tbsp plain flour
1 tsp ground cinnamon
300ml (½ pint) chicken stock
300ml (½ pint) low-fat natural yogurt
2 tbsp chopped fresh coriander
salt and freshly ground black pepper, to taste

1 Heat a non-stick frying pan and dry-fry the onion until
   soft. Add the garlic and the chicken and cook for 2–3
   minutes until the chicken changes colour.
2 Sprinkle the curry powder and flour over the chicken.
   Toss the chicken so that it is completely covered, then
   add the cinnamon and cook for 1 minute.
3 Gradually add the stock, stirring well, and season to taste
   with salt and black pepper. Simmer gently for 10 minutes
   until the sauce thickens.
4 Remove the pan from the heat, stir in the yogurt and
   coriander and serve immediately.

Chicken Tikka Masala

Per serving 245 calories 2% fat
Serves 2 Prep time 10 mins Cook time 30 mins

2 × 120g skinless chicken breasts, cut into chunks
200g pouch Rosemary Conley Low-Fat Tikka Masala Sauce
1 tbsp 2% fat Greek yogurt
freshly ground black pepper, to taste
fresh coriander, to serve

1 Heat a non-stick frying pan and dry-fry the chicken until
   lightly browned. Stir in the tikka masala sauce and
   simmer gently for 20 minutes until the chicken is cooked.
2 Just before serving, remove from heat, stir in the yogurt
   and sprinkle with chopped coriander.

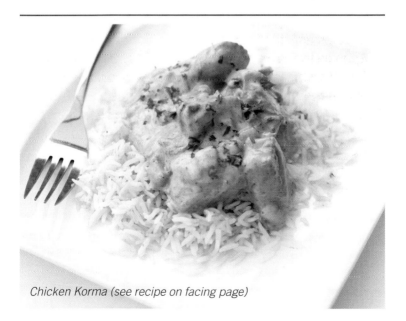

Chicken Korma (see recipe on facing page)

Cajun Chicken Casserole

Per serving 256 calories 2.9% fat
Serves 4 Prep time 10 mins Cook time 40 mins

8 skinless chicken thighs
1 tbsp Cajun spice
1 large red onion, diced
2 garlic cloves, crushed
1 red pepper, finely diced
500g tomato passata
salt and freshly ground black pepper, to taste

1 Preheat the oven to 200°C, 400°F, Gas Mark 6.
2 Arrange the chicken thighs in the base of an ovenproof
   dish, sprinkle with the Cajun spice and season with salt
   and black pepper. Cover with the onion, garlic and red
   pepper.
3 Cover the dish, then bake in the oven for 10 minutes.
   Remove from the oven and pour the passata over the
   chicken. Return the dish to the oven for a further 30
   minutes. Serve hot or cold.

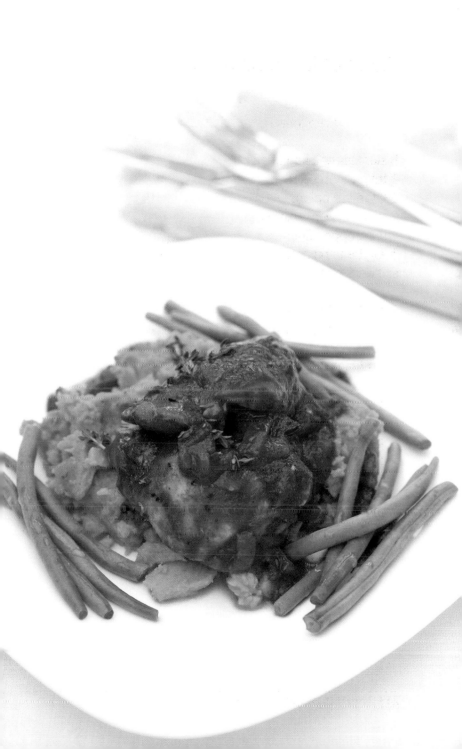

Fennel Jerk Chicken

Per serving 102 calories 1% fat
Serves 4 Prep time 10 mins Cook time 30 mins

2 large skinless chicken breasts
1 tsp smoked paprika
1 tbsp jerk seasoning
zest and juice of 1 orange

2 garlic cloves, crushed
1 head fennel, sliced
salt and freshly ground
black pepper, to taste

1 Preheat a large non-stick frying pan.
2 Slice the chicken into pieces, then place in a bowl with
   the paprika, jerk seasoning, garlic, orange zest and juice
   and fennel and mix well.
3 When the pan is hot, add the chicken and cook for about
   30 minutes, stirring well and moving it around the pan to
   ensure even cooking.
4 To check if the chicken is cooked, insert a knife into the
   thickest part of the flesh. If the juices run clear, the
   chicken is ready.

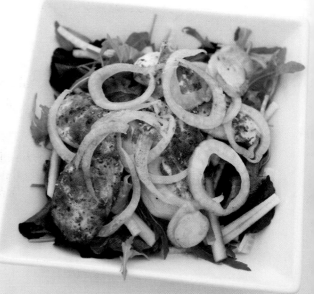

Oven-Baked Chicken Tikka Masala

Per serving 249 calories 0.8% fat
Serves 4 Prep time 5 mins (plus marinating time)
Cook time 35 mins

4 skinless chicken breasts
600ml (1 pint) tomato passata
300ml (½ pint) low-fat natural yogurt
2 tbsp chopped fresh coriander
salt and freshly ground black pepper, to taste
mint leaves, to garnish

for the tikka paste
1 small red onion
4 tbsp tomato purée
1 tsp ground cumin
½ tsp ground cinnamon
2.5cm piece fresh ginger, grated
2 garlic cloves, crushed
1 small red chilli, deseeded and chopped
juice of 1 lime
2 tsp vegetable stock powder

1 Preheat the oven to 200°C, 400°F, Gas Mark 6. Cut the
   chicken into chunks, place in a bowl and season well
   with salt and black pepper.
2 Place all the tikka paste ingredients in a food processor
   or blender and blend until smooth. Spread the tikka
   paste mixture over the chicken pieces, coating them on
   all sides. Leave in a cool place to marinate for 20
   minutes.

continued…

3 Transfer the chicken to a non-stick roasting tin and cook in the oven for 15 minutes until lightly roasted.
4 Remove from the oven and stir in the passata. Return to the oven for a further 10 minutes to heat through. Just before serving, stir in the yogurt and coriander. Spoon into warmed serving dishes and garnish with mint leaves.

Honey and Mustard Chicken

Per serving 253 calories 2.1% fat
Serves 2 Prep time 10 mins Cook time 25–30 mins

2 × 150g skinless chicken breasts
2 tbsp soft set honey
2 tbsp grain mustard
1 tbsp white balsamic dressing or white wine vinegar
salt and freshly ground black pepper, to taste
chopped fresh chives, to garnish

1 Preheat the oven to 200°C, 400°F, Gas Mark 6.
2 Using a sharp knife, make several incisions along the top of each chicken breast and season with salt and black pepper.
3 Mix together the honey, mustard and balsamic dressing or vinegar and pour over the chicken breasts.
4 Place the chicken on a non-stick baking tray and bake in the centre of the oven for 25–30 minutes, until cooked through. Transfer to serving plates and garnish with the chopped chives. Serve hot or cold.

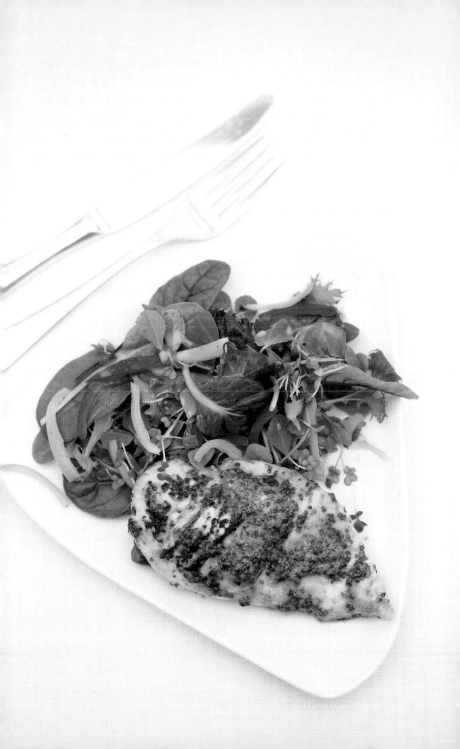

Spicy Baked Chicken with Parsnips

Per serving 253 calories 4.2% fat
Serves 4 Prep time 10 mins (plus marinating time)
Cook time 30–35 mins

4 chicken thighs, skin removed
4 parsnips, peeled and cut into chunks

for the marinade
1 red onion, finely diced
1 garlic clove, crushed
1 tsp ground coriander
2 tbsp reduced-salt soy sauce
zest and juice of 1 lime
1 small red chilli, chopped
1 tbsp tomato purée

1 Preheat the oven to 200°C, 400°F, Gas Mark 6.
2 Mix all the marinade ingredients together (this can be done in a blender for ease).
3 Place the chicken pieces in a shallow dish with the parsnips and pour the marinade over. Leave to marinate for at least 30 minutes.
4 Remove the chicken pieces and parsnips to a non-stick oven tray and bake for 30–35 minutes, turning regularly to ensure even cooking.
5 To check if the chicken is cooked, insert a knife into the thickest part of the flesh. If the juices run clear, the chicken is ready. Serve with the parsnips.

Easy Jerk Barbecue Chicken

Per serving 339 calories 5.3% fat
Serves 2 Prep time 10 mins (plus marinating time)
Cook time 35 mins

2 small chicken thighs, skin removed
1 red onion, finely sliced
100g chestnut mushrooms, cut into quarters
200g pouch Rosemary Conley Low-Fat Jerk
   Barbecue Sauce
salad leaves, to serve

1 Place the chicken thighs in an ovenproof dish. Cover with
   the onion and mushrooms, then drizzle the jerk
   barbecue sauce over. Using 2 forks, turn the chicken
   and vegetables to coat them well. Leave to marinate for
   30 minutes.
2 Meanwhile, preheat the oven to 200°C, 400°F, Gas
   Mark 6.
3 When ready to cook, bake the chicken in the oven for
   35 minutes until the chicken is fully cooked. Serve with
   salad leaves.

Chicken Liver Pasta

Per serving 248 calories 1.2% fat
Serves 4 Prep time 10 mins Cooking time 20 mins

180g (dry weight) pasta
1 vegetable stock cube
1 red onion, finely diced
1 garlic clove, crushed
225g chicken livers
pinch of dried chilli flakes
1 tbsp chopped fresh basil
200ml tomato passata
salt and freshly ground black pepper, to taste
fresh basil, to garnish

1 Preheat the oven to 200°C, 400°F, Gas Mark 6.
2 Cook the pasta in a pan of boiling water with the stock
  cube.
3 Meanwhile, heat a large non-stick pan and dry-fry the
  diced onion and crushed garlic for 3–4 minutes until soft.
  Add the chicken livers and cook for 1 minute to seal
  them, then stir in the chilli, basil and passata and bring
  the sauce to a gentle simmer.
4 Drain the pasta and season with salt and black pepper.
  Divide between 4 serving bowls and top with the sauce.
  Just before serving, garnish with basil.

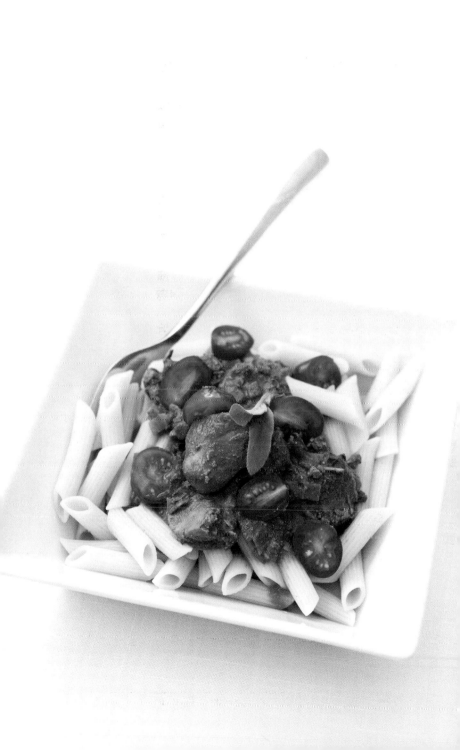

Jerk Chicken and Potato Bake

Per serving 220 calories 1% fat
Serves 4 Prep time 10 mins Cook time 25 mins

4 skinless chicken breasts, diced
1 tbsp jerk paste
1 large red onion, finely diced
2 garlic cloves, crushed
300g cooked new potatoes, sliced
200ml semi-skimmed milk
salt and freshly ground black pepper, to taste

1 Preheat the oven to 200°C, 400°F, Gas Mark 6.
2 Place the diced chicken in a mixing bowl. Add the jerk
   paste, red onion, garlic and sliced potatoes, then
   combine well and season with salt and black pepper.
3 Spoon the chicken and potato into the base of an
   ovenproof dish. Pour the milk over
   the mixture and bake
   for 25 minutes.
   Serve hot.

Thai Red Chicken Curry

Per serving 264 calories 0.8% fat
Serves 2 Prep time 25 mins Cook time 30 mins

1 red onion, diced
1 garlic clove, chopped
2 skinless chicken breasts, diced
1 red pepper, deseeded and finely diced
200g pouch Rosemary Conley Low-Fat Thai Red Sauce
1 tsp arrowroot
1 tbsp chopped fresh basil
salt and freshly ground black pepper, to taste

1 Heat a non-stick wok or frying pan and dry-fry the onion and garlic until soft and lightly coloured. Add the chicken and seal the outside of the meat, seasoning with salt and black pepper.
2 Add the red pepper and continue cooking for 2 minutes before adding the sauce.
3 Mix the arrowroot with a little cold water. Reduce the heat and allow to simmer, stirring in the arrowroot gently as the sauce thickens. Adjust the consistency with a little hot water. Just before serving, stir in the basil.

Turkey Spaghetti

Per serving 253 calories 1.9% fat
Serves 4 Prep time 10 mins Cook time 35 mins

200g lean minced turkey
100g mushrooms, finely sliced
2 garlic cloves, crushed
1 red onion, finely chopped
1 red pepper, deseeded and finely diced
400g tin chopped tomatoes
1 tbsp tomato purée
pinch of freeze-dried Italian herbs
1 tsp vegetable stock powder
100g (dry weight) spaghetti
1 vegetable stock cube
fresh basil, to serve
10g fresh Parmesan, to serve (optional)

1 Heat a non-stick pan and dry-fry the turkey mince until
   lightly browned. Add the mushrooms, garlic and red
   onion and pepper, and lightly cook until soft.
2 Stir in the tinned tomatoes, tomato purée, herbs and
   stock powder, mixing well. Simmer gently for 30 minutes
   until the meat is tender.
3 Meanwhile, cook the spaghetti in a pan of boiling water
   with the vegetable stock cube added. Drain, then
   transfer to serving plates, pour the sauce on top and
   sprinkle with fresh basil and Parmesan (if using).

Roast Turkey Leg Fricassee

Per serving 238 calories 1.6% fat
Serves 4 Prep time 10 mins Cook time 1 hr 20 mins

1 turkey leg on the bone (approx. 900g weighed with bone)
2 medium onions, finely chopped
2 garlic cloves, crushed
1 tsp chopped fresh thyme
1 tbsp flour
1 tsp ground turmeric
1 tbsp chicken stock
2 tbsp sherry
200g chestnut mushrooms, sliced
300ml (½ pint) semi-skimmed milk
salt and freshly ground black pepper, to taste

1 Preheat the oven to 200°C, 400°F, Gas Mark 6.
2 Place the turkey leg in a roasting tin and cook, uncovered, for 1 hour. When cooked, remove the turkey from the oven, strip the meat from the bone and cut into pieces.
3 Heat a non-stick wok or frying pan and dry-fry the onions and garlic until soft. Stir in the thyme, flour and turmeric and cook out for 1 minute, before stirring in the chicken stock and sherry. Now add the mushrooms, then stir in the milk and roast turkey meat and bring the sauce to a gentle simmer for 10 minutes, to allow it to thicken. Check the seasoning and serve straight away.

Crispy Turkey Escalopes with Noodles

Per serving 303 calories 2% fat
Serves 2 Prep time 5 mins Cook time 20 mins

low-cal oil spray, for frying
1 egg
2 × 100g thin turkey escalopes
2 tbsp bramata polenta flour
200g cooked noodles
8 cherry tomatoes
2 tsp balsamic jelly
salt and freshly ground black pepper, to taste

1 Preheat a non-stick frying pan and add a little oil spray.
  Beat the egg in a shallow dish, adding salt and black
  pepper. Dip the turkey escalopes in the egg and then in
  the polenta flour.
2 Add the noodles to the dish with the beaten egg and
  leave until ready to cook.
3 Cook the coated turkey steaks in the hot pan for 5–6
  minutes on each side, then remove them from the pan
  and keep warm.
4 Add the noodles to the pan and cook for 3 minutes on
  each side.
5 Cut the tomatoes in half and mix with the balsamic jelly
  in a bowl.
6 Serve the turkey on a bed of salad with the noodles and
  the tomato salad.

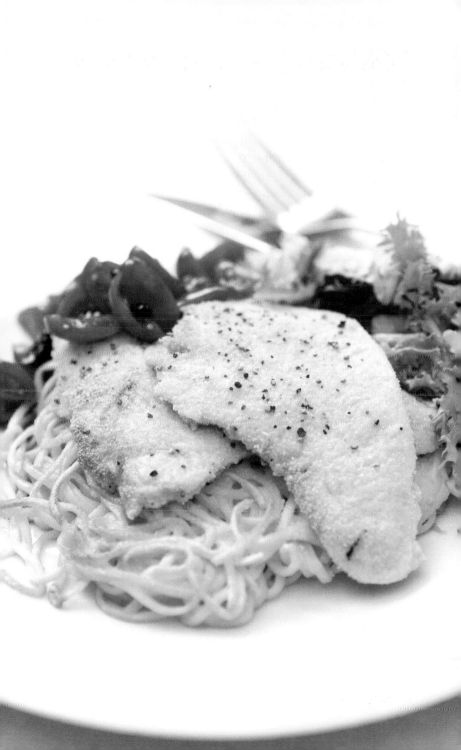

Mushroom and Turkey Noodles

Per serving 199 calories 0.6% fat
Serves 4 Prep time 10 mins Cook time 10 mins

400g thin turkey steaks, sliced
1 garlic clove, crushed
200g pack stir-fry vegetables
100g pak choi, sliced
250g chestnut mushrooms, sliced
2 tsp reduced-salt soy sauce
1 tsp rice vinegar
2 tbsp mango chutney
squeeze of fresh lemon juice
300g cooked noodles
freshly ground black pepper, to taste
chilli sauce, to serve

1 Heat a non-stick wok and dry-fry the turkey steaks and
   garlic for 3–4 minutes over a high heat, seasoning with
   plenty of black pepper.
2 Add the stir-fry vegetables, pak choi and mushrooms and
   cook for a further 1–2 minutes. Add the remaining
   ingredients, including the cooked noodles, and toss well
   together. Serve straight away with a little chilli sauce.

Fish and Shellfish

Smoked Mackerel Pâté

Per serving 165 calories 19.5% fat
Serves 6 Prep time 10 mins

This recipe is allowed on my FAB Diet despite the high fat content because of the health benefits of oily fish.

250g smoked mackerel fillets
1 tbsp horseradish sauce
1 tsp grain mustard
2 tbsp 2% fat Greek yogurt
4 spring onions, finely chopped
1 tbsp lime juice
salt and freshly ground black pepper, to taste

1 Using a fork, break the fish away from the skin and into a bowl. Add the spring onions, horseradish sauce, mustard, lime juice and yogurt, mix well and season with black pepper and salt if required.
2 Press the mixture into ramekins or serving pots and chill until required. (Once made, this pâté will keep for up to 5 days in the fridge, or it can be stored in the freezer until required.)

Sardine Tagliatelle

Per serving 260 calories 1.9% fat
Serves 4 Prep time 5 mins Cook time 20 mins

200g (dry weight) tagliatelle pasta
1 vegetable stock cube
2 baby leeks, finely chopped
1 garlic clove, crushed
120g tin sardines in tomato sauce
400g tin chopped tomatoes
1 tsp vegetable stock powder
1 tbsp chopped fresh basil, plus extra to garnish
salt and freshly ground black pepper, to taste
cherry tomatoes, to garnish

1 Cook the pasta in a large pan of boiling water containing
   the stock cube.
2 Meanwhile, heat a separate non-stick pan and dry-fry the
   leeks and garlic until soft. Stir in the sardines, chopped
   tomatoes and stock powder and simmer to allow the
   tomatoes to reduce. Season with salt and black pepper to
   taste, then the 1 tablespoon of basil and reduce the heat.
3 Drain the pasta and transfer to serving bowls. Remove
   the sauce from the heat and spoon over the pasta. Serve
   garnished with cherry tomatoes and extra fresh basil.

Chinese Salmon Steaks with Stir-Fried Vegetables

Per serving 414 calories 4.8% fat
Serves 2 Prep time 15 mins Cook time 15 mins

2 salmon steaks
2 tsp finely grated lemon zest
2 tsp garlic sauce
1 tbsp sweet chilli sauce
310g pack beansprouts
100g watercress
150ml pineapple juice
salt and freshly ground black pepper, to taste

1 Preheat the oven to 200°C, 400°F, Gas Mark 6.
2 Place the salmon steaks on a non-stick baking tray and
   season on both sides with salt and black pepper.
3 In a small bowl, mix together the lemon zest, garlic sauce
   and chilli sauce and then drizzle it over the steaks.
4 Bake the steaks in the oven for 8–10 minutes until just
   cooked.
5 Meanwhile, heat a non-stick wok or frying pan and, just
   before the salmon is cooked, stir-fry the beansprouts and
   watercress until just wilted, adding the pineapple juice.
6 Transfer the wilted vegetables to serving plates and top
   with the salmon steaks. Serve hot or cold.

Salmon with Spiced Cucumber

Per serving 221 calories 5.6% fat
Serves 4 Prep time 5 mins Cook time 10–15 mins

1 cucumber, peeled and cut into sticks
1 red pepper, deseeded and sliced
4 salmon fillets
zest and juice of 1 lime
2 tbsp Thai sweet chilli dipping sauce
2 tsp palm sugar (or honey or maple syrup)
salt and freshly ground black pepper, to taste
lime wedges and fresh herbs, to garnish

1 Preheat the oven to 200°C, 400°F, Gas Mark 6.
2 Put the cucumber and red pepper in the base of a non-stick roasting pan. Arrange the salmon fillets on top and season with salt and black pepper. Sprinkle a little lime zest and juice on top of each fillet, then dot with chilli sauce and palm sugar.
3 Bake, uncovered, for 10–15 minutes, until the salmon is just cooked. Transfer the steaks to serving plates and garnish with fresh herbs and lime wedges.

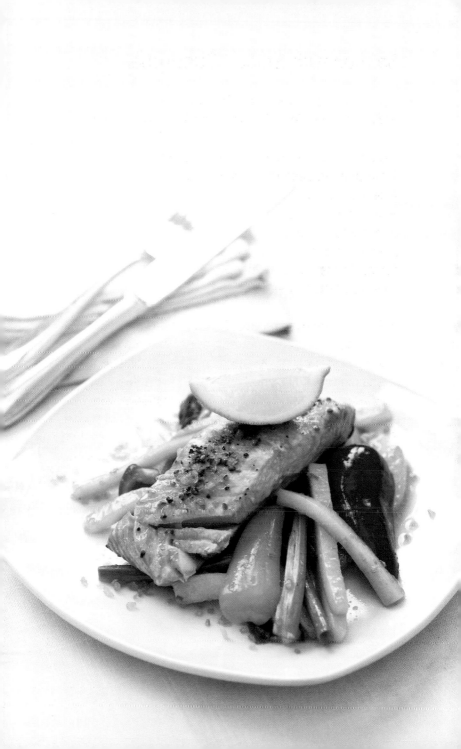

Tandoori Salmon with Spicy Noodles

Per serving 383 calories 6.5% fat
Serves 2 Prep time 5 mins Cook time 10 mins

2 salmon steaks
2 tsp tandoori curry powder
200g cooked rice noodles
2 tbsp spicy Szechuan sauce
salt and freshly ground black pepper, to taste

1 Preheat the oven to 200°C, 400°F, Gas Mark 6.
2 Roll the salmon steaks in the curry powder and season
   with salt and black pepper, then place on a non-stick
   baking tray. Bake in the oven for 6–8 minutes until just
   cooked.
3 Meanwhile heat a non-stick pan and stir-fry the noodles
   with the sauce until heated through. Serve the salmon on
   a bed of noodles.

Salmon Fish Fingers

Per serving 235 calories 7.6% fat
Serves 4 Prep time 10 mins Cook time 15 mins

300g salmon fillet
100g coarse polenta flour
3 tbsp Hellmann's extra-light mayonnaise
1 garlic clove, crushed
1 tsp ground coriander
1 small red chilli, finely chopped
2 tbsp chopped fresh coriander, to serve
salt and black pepper, to taste

1 Preheat the oven to 200°C, 400°F, Gas Mark 6.
2 Cut the salmon into strips and place in a shallow bowl.
   Season with salt and black pepper then roll the strips in
   the polenta flour, coating all sides. Place on a non-stick
   baking tray and bake in the oven for 15 minutes.
3 In a small bowl, mix together the mayonnaise, garlic,
   ground coriander and chilli.
4 Transfer the salmon fish fingers to serving plates,
   sprinkle with fresh coriander and serve with the
   coriander mayonnaise.

Tikka Salmon

Per serving 328 calories 4.6% fat
Serves 2 Prep time 10 mins (plus marinating time)
Cook time 20 mins

2 × 120g salmon steaks
200g pouch Rosemary Conley Low-Fat Tikka Masala Sauce
1 red onion, diced
200g baby leaf spinach, shredded
freshly ground black pepper, to taste

1 Place the salmon in a bowl. Pour the tikka masala sauce over the salmon, coating it well, and leave to marinate for at least 30 minutes.
2 Heat a non-stick pan and dry-fry the onion until lightly coloured. Add the salmon and tikka masala sauce and bring to a gentle simmer. Simmer for 8–10 minutes.
3 Just before serving, remove the salmon and stir in the spinach, seasoning with some freshly ground black pepper.

Arrabbiata Prawns

Per serving 113 calories 0.4% fat
Serves 2 Prep time 10 mins Cook time 20 mins

120g uncooked prawns
1 red onion, finely chopped
1 garlic clove, crushed
200g pouch Rosemary Conley Low-Fat Tomato
    and Chilli Sauce
1 tbsp 0% fat Greek yogurt
salt and freshly ground black pepper, to taste
fresh coriander, to serve

1 Rinse the prawns well under cold running water.
2 Heat a non-stick frying pan and dry-fry the onion for 2–3
   minutes until soft, then add the garlic and cook for a
   further minute.
3 Stir in the tomato and chilli sauce and bring to a gentle
   simmer. Add the prawns and allow to heat through.
4 Remove the pan from the heat and stir in the yogurt.
   Season to taste with salt and black pepper, stir in the
   coriander and serve straight away.

Sweet Chilli Prawns

Per serving 95 calories 0.6% fat
Serves 4 Prep time 5 mins Cook time 20 mins

1 red onion, finely chopped
2 garlic cloves, crushed
2 tbsp sweet chilli sauce
400g tin chopped tomatoes
2 tsp lime pickle
225g fresh uncooked peeled prawns
freshly ground black pepper, to taste
1 tbsp chopped fresh coriander, to serve

1 Heat a heavy-based, non-stick pan, then add the onion
   and dry-fry until soft. Add the garlic and cook for 1
   minute, then stir in the chilli sauce, tomatoes and lime
   pickle and bring to a gentle simmer.
2 Add the prawns and cook until they firm up and change
   colour. Just before serving, stir in the chopped coriander.

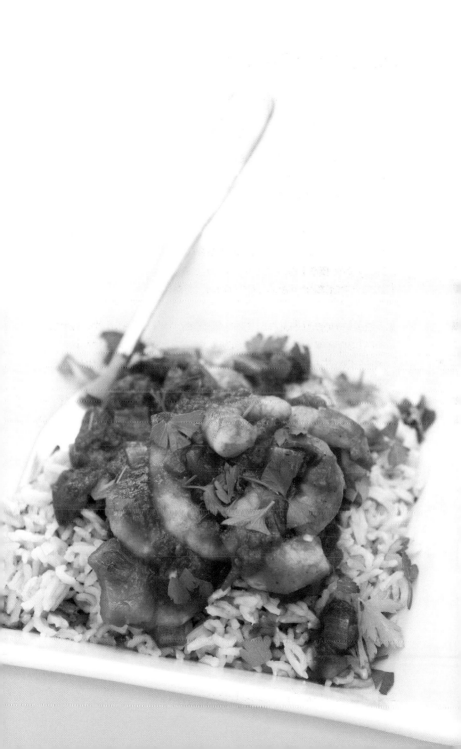

Coconut Prawns

Per serving 206 calories 1.5% fat
Serves 2 Prep time 5 mins Cook time 10 mins

1 red onion, chopped
220g raw peeled prawns
150g stir-fry asparagus
1 chilli coconut shot stir-fry sauce
1 tbsp 2% fat Greek yogurt

1 Heat a non-stick pan and dry-fry the onion until soft. Add the prawns and asparagus along with the stir-fry sauce, and simmer gently for about 10 minutes, until the prawns are cooked through.
2 Just before serving, remove from the heat and stir in the yogurt.

Seared Tuna with Chilli Cream

Per serving 153 calories 4% fat
Serves 4 Prep time 10 mins Cook time 20 mins

olive oil spray, for frying
4 tuna steaks (approx. 100g each)
salt and freshly ground black pepper

for the dressing
2 tbsp 2% fat Greek yogurt
1 garlic clove, crushed
1 small red chilli, deseeded and finely chopped

1 Preheat a non-stick griddle pan and lightly spray with oil
   spray. Season the tuna steaks with salt and black pepper,
   add to the hot pan and cook until the colour changes
   halfway up the sides of the steaks. Turn them over and
   cook on the other side, then remove from the pan and
   allow to rest for 1–2 minutes.
2 Mix together the dressing ingredients and season with
   salt and black pepper.
3 Spoon the dressing over the tuna steaks and serve
   straight away.

Smoked Fish Laksa

Per serving 192 calories 0.6% fat
Serves 4 Prep time 10 mins Cook time 20 mins

2 onions, chopped
2 garlic cloves, crushed
600ml (1 pint) vegetable stock
2 tbsp plain flour
½ tsp ground turmeric
600ml (1 pint) skimmed milk
320g mixed diced fish (e.g. smoked haddock and cod)
salt and freshly ground black pepper, to taste
2 tbsp chopped fresh parsley, to serve

1 Heat a large non-stick pan and dry-fry the onions and garlic for 1–2 minutes until soft. Stir in 3 tablespoons of the vegetable stock and then mix in the flour and turmeric. Cook for 1 minute, then stir in the remaining stock and the skimmed milk and bring to a gentle simmer to allow the mixture to thicken.
2 When the mixture has thickened, add the fish and continue to cook for a further 4–5 minutes. Season with salt and black pepper to taste. Just before serving, stir in the parsley.

Top: Smoked Fish Laksa
Bottom: Red Pepper Houmous Baked Cod
(for recipe see page 248)

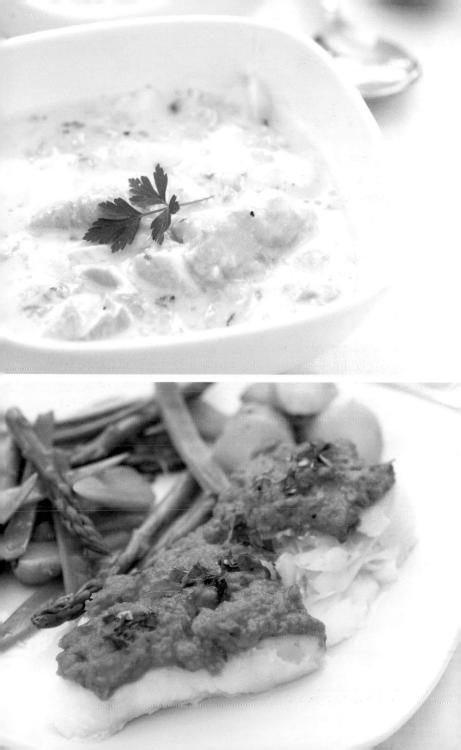

Red Pepper Houmous Baked Cod

Per serving 140 calories 1.2% fat
Serves 4 Prep time 15 mins Cook time 15–20 mins

450g thick cod fillet
½ red pepper, chopped
130g tin chickpeas, drained
2 garlic cloves, crushed
1 tsp vegetable stock powder
3 tsp lemon juice
about 50ml boiling water
freshly ground black pepper

1 Preheat the oven to 200°C, 400°F, Gas Mark 6, and
   preheat a non-stick frying pan.
2 Cut the cod into 4 equal-sized pieces and place in an
   ovenproof dish.
3 To make the houmous, dry-fry the red pepper in the hot
   pan until soft. Transfer to a blender, add the chickpeas,
   garlic, stock powder and lemon juice and a little boiling
   water (no more than 50ml) and blend until you have a
   smooth paste.
4 Spread the paste over the fish and bake in the oven for
   10–15 minutes. Allow to rest for 1 minute before serving.

Illustrated on page 247 (bottom)

Thai Cod Laksa

Per serving 111 calories 0.7% fat
Serves 2 Prep time 10 mins Cook time 20 mins

1 onion, sliced
1 garlic clove, crushed
300ml (½ pint) vegetable stock
1 tbsp plain flour
200g pouch Rosemary Conley Low-Fat Thai Red Sauce
100g fresh cod, diced
salt and freshly ground black pepper, to taste
1 tbsp chopped fresh parsley, to serve

1 Heat a large non-stick pan and dry-fry the onions and
   garlic for 1–2 minutes until soft. Add 3 tablespoons of the
   vegetable stock, then sprinkle over the flour and mix in.
   Cook for 1 minute then stir in the remaining stock and
   the Thai Red Sauce, bring to a gentle simmer and cook
   for 2–3 minutes. Add the cod and cook for 2 minutes
   more.
2 Adjust the seasoning with salt and black pepper. Just
   before serving stir in the parsley.

Seafood with Black Rice Noodles

Per serving 195 calories 1.4% fat
Serves 4 Prep time 10 mins Cook time 10 mins

140g (dry weight) black rice noodles
1 vegetable stock cube
2 onions, finely chopped
2 garlic cloves, crushed
300g prepared mixed seafood
60ml rosé wine
1 tsp vegetable stock powder
2 tbsp 2% fat Greek yogurt
freshly ground black pepper, to taste
1 tbsp chopped fresh parsley, to garnish

1 Cook the rice noodles in a pan of boiling water with the
   vegetable stock cube.
2 Meanwhile, heat a non-stick wok and dry-fry the
   chopped onions and garlic over a medium heat for 2–3
   minutes, seasoning well with black pepper.
3 Add the seafood and wine and heat for 1–2 minutes to
   reduce the wine, then remove the pan from the heat and
   stir in the stock powder and yogurt.
4 Drain the noodles and arrange on serving plates. Top
   with the seafood and garnish with the parsley.

Vegetarian

Aubergine and Artichoke Gratin ⊙

Per serving 90 calories 0.6% fat
Serves 4 Prep time 15 mins Cook time 10 mins

1 large aubergine, diced
2 leeks, diced
2 garlic cloves, crushed
100g mushrooms, finely chopped
1 red chilli, chopped
200g tinned artichoke pieces
1 tsp vegetable stock powder
30g fresh breadcrumbs
30g grated low-fat mature cheese (max. 5% fat)

1 Preheat the oven to 200°C, 400°F, Gas Mark 6.
2 Heat a non-stick pan and dry-fry the aubergine, leeks
   and garlic until soft. Stir in the mushrooms and cook until
   the mixture starts to colour, then add the chilli,
   artichokes and stock powder and continue to simmer for
   10 minutes.
3 Spoon the mixture into an ovenproof dish and sprinkle
   the breadcrumbs and cheese over the top. Bake in the
   oven for 10 minutes until brown on top.

Bombay Potatoes ⊘

Per serving 129 calories 0.4% fat
Serves 4 (as a side dish) Prep time 5 mins
Cook time 25 mins

1 red onion, chopped
2 garlic cloves, crushed
500g new potatoes, washed and diced
1 red pepper, diced
1 tbsp fajita paste
20g low-fat mature cheese (max. 5% fat), grated
1 tbsp chopped fresh parsley, to garnish

1 Heat a non-stick pan and dry-fry the onion and garlic until soft.
2 Add the potatoes and red pepper. Pour over enough boiling water to cover the vegetables, then mix in the fajita paste. Simmer gently until the potatoes are cooked and most of the liquid has reduced. Serve sprinkled with the grated cheese and fresh parsley.

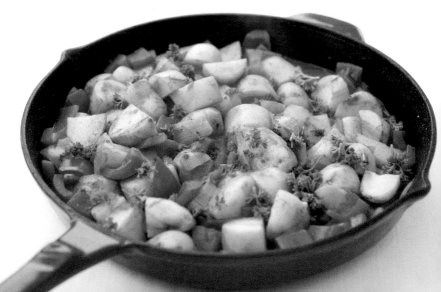

Vegetable Biryani ✅

Per serving 172 calories 0.8% fat
Serves 4 Prep time 10 mins Cook time 25 mins

1 small red onion, finely chopped
1 celery stick, finely sliced
1 small red pepper, deseeded and finely diced
225g chestnut mushrooms, sliced
1 courgette, diced
1 garlic clove, crushed
100g (dry weight) basmati rice
600ml (1 pint) vegetable stock
400g tin chopped tomatoes
pinch of saffron strands
1 tsp chopped fresh thyme
100g frozen peas
50g frozen sweetcorn
salt and freshly ground black pepper, to taste

1 Heat a non-stick wok and dry-fry the onion, celery, pepper, courgette, mushrooms and garlic over a high heat for 4–5 minutes, stirring occasionally.
2 Add the rice, vegetable stock, tomatoes, saffron and thyme. Stir well and then simmer gently for about 20 minutes to allow the liquid to be absorbed. Check the seasoning, adding salt and pepper to taste.
3 Just before serving, stir in the frozen peas and sweetcorn and heat through before serving. Serve hot or cold.

Crushed Bean Rigatoni ✓

Per serving 280 calories 3% fat
Serves 4 Prep time 20 mins Cook time 30 mins

200g rigatoni pasta tubes
1 vegetable stock cube
200g frozen baby broad beans
1 tbsp chopped fresh mint
100g extra-light soft cheese with chives
2 tbsp 2% fat Greek yogurt
1 tbsp chopped fresh parsley
2 tsp capers

1 Cook the pasta in a pan of boiling water containing the
   stock cube.
2 Meanwhile, in a separate saucepan, boil the beans until
   soft. Drain and mash with a potato masher, removing as
   many skins as possible.
3 Drain the pasta and return to the pan, add the beans and
   the remaining ingredients and mix well. Spoon into
   serving dishes.

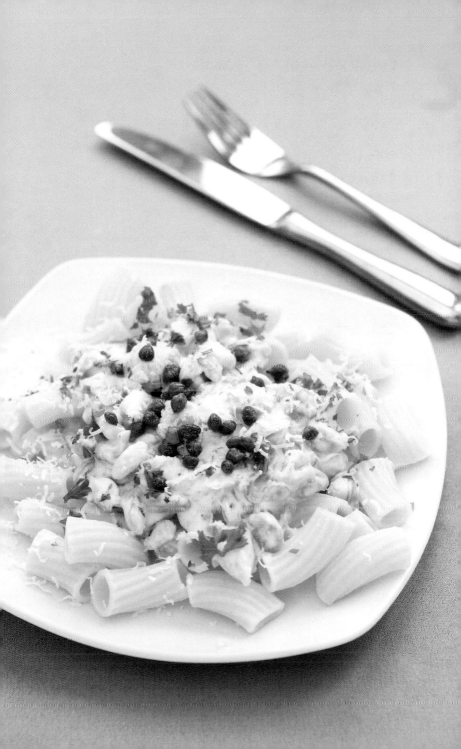

Tomato Risotto with Roasted Vegetables ✔

Per serving 271 calories 0.4% fat
Serves 4 Prep time 5 mins Cook time 35 mins

for the roasted vegetables
2 courgettes, sliced
2 red peppers, cut into chunks
1 red onion, sliced into wedges
32 cherry tomatoes

1 tbsp balsamic vinegar,
    plus more to serve
oil spray, for frying

for the risotto
1 onion, finely chopped
1 garlic clove, crushed
200g Arborio risotto rice
400g tin chopped tomatoes
600ml (1 pint) vegetable stock

1 tbsp chopped fresh
    parsley
salt and freshly ground
    black pepper, to taste

1 Preheat the oven to 200°C, 400°F, Gas Mark 6.
2 Place the roasting vegetables on a non-stick baking tray
   and lightly spray with oil spray. Drizzle with balsamic
   vinegar and bake in the oven for 15 minutes or until
   lightly charred.
3 To prepare the risotto, heat a non-stick pan and dry-fry
   the onion and garlic until soft. Add the rice and tomatoes
   and then gradually stir in the vegetable stock, allowing
   the rice to absorb it before adding more – this will take
   15–20 minutes.
4 Once all the liquid has been added, stir in the chopped
   parsley. Season with salt and black pepper to taste. Serve
   the roasted vegetables and risotto in warmed bowls
   drizzled with a little extra balsamic vinegar.

Swiss Chard Lasagne ⊘

Per serving 241 calories 1.7% fat
Serves 6 Prep time 20 mins Cook time 20 mins

500ml semi-skimmed milk
4 tsp cornflour
1 tsp mustard powder
100g extra-light soft cheese
1 tsp vegetable stock powder
6 sheets fresh lasagne
300g Swiss chard leaves
30g low-fat mature cheese (max. 5% fat), grated

1 Preheat the oven to 200°C, 400°F, Gas Mark 6.
2 Reserve a little cold milk to mix with the cornflour, and
   heat the remainder in a saucepan. Mix the cornflour with
   the cold milk and whisk into the hot milk, then continue
   whisking to allow the sauce to thicken. Stir in the
   mustard powder, extra-light soft cheese and stock
   powder.
3 Blanch the pasta sheets in a large pan of boiling water for
   2 minutes, then remove and allow to drain individually on
   a tray. Add the chard to the water and wilt for 30
   seconds, then drain well.
4 Assemble the lasagne by placing alternate layers of
   chard, sauce and pasta in an ovenproof dish, finishing
   with a layer of sauce. Top with the grated cheese and
   bake in the oven for 20 minutes until golden brown.

Illustrated on page 258 (bottom)

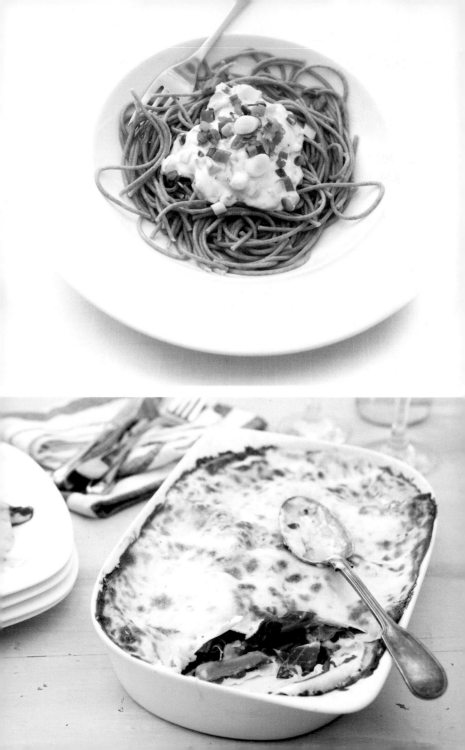

Garlic Mushroom Spelt Spaghetti ⓥ

Per serving 252 calories 2% fat
Serves 4 Prep time 5 mins Cook time 20 mins

180g spelt spaghetti
1 vegetable stock cube
2 garlic cloves, chopped
100ml white wine
200g chestnut mushrooms, sliced
juice of 1 lime
200g extra-light cream cheese
4 spring onions, finely chopped
freshly ground black pepper, to taste
fresh basil, to garnish

1 Cook the pasta in a large pan of boiling water with the vegetable stock cube.
2 Meanwhile, heat a separate non-stick pan and dry-fry the garlic for 1–2 minutes. Add the wine and mushrooms and cook over a moderate heat, adding the lime juice and black pepper to taste. Stir in the cheese and heat through.
3 Drain the pasta and divide between 4 warmed serving plates.
4 Add the spring onions to the sauce, stir well, then spoon the sauce over the pasta. Serve garnished with fresh basil.

Top: Garlic Mushroom Spelt Spaghetti
Bottom: Swiss Chard Lasagne (see recipe on page 257)

Roasted Vegetable Pasta with Garlic Bread ✅

Per serving 353 calories 1.6% fat
  (including 1 slice garlic bread)
Serves 2 Prep time 10 mins Cook time 25 mins

400g roasting vegetables (e.g. peppers, onions,
    courgettes, aubergine)
100g wholewheat pasta shapes
1 vegetable stock cube
1 tsp low-fat pesto
oil spray, for roasting
salt and freshly ground black pepper, to taste

for the garlic bread
1 small baguette
1 tbsp extra-light mayonnaise
1 garlic clove, crushed
pinch of ground turmeric

1 Preheat the oven to 200°C, 400°F, Gas Mark 6.
2 Place the vegetables in a roasting tin and lightly spray
    with oil spray and season with salt and black pepper.
    Roast in the oven for 20 minutes.
3 Meanwhile cook the pasta in a pan of boiling water with
    the vegetable stock cube.
4 Make the garlic bread by cutting the baguette lengthways
    into 2 slices and place on a non-stick baking tray. In a
    small bowl mix together the mayonnaise, garlic and
    turmeric and spread it over the bread. Five minutes
    before serving, put the bread in the oven for 5 minutes.

5 Drain the pasta well, then return it to the pan and stir in the pesto. Add the roasted vegetables and mix well. Spoon into serving bowls and serve with the garlic bread.

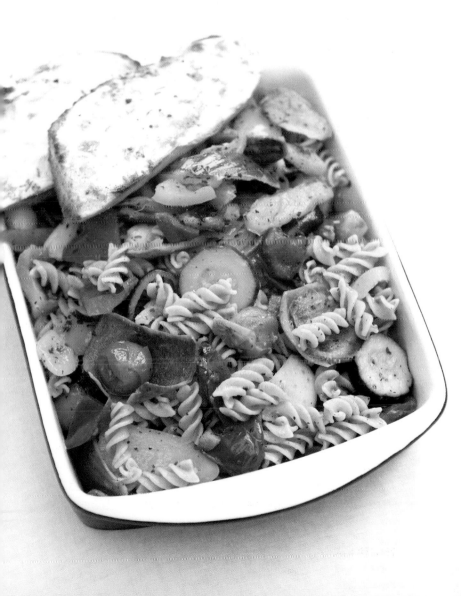

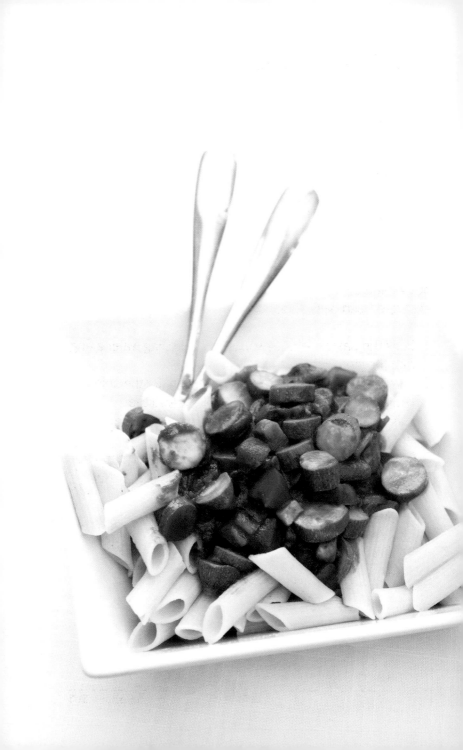

Baby Courgette Pasta ✔

Per serving 234 calories 0.6% fat
Serves 4 Prep time 5 mins Cook time 20 mins

180g (dry weight) pasta shapes
1 vegetable stock cube
1 small red onion, finely sliced
2 garlic cloves, crushed
250g baby courgettes, chopped
1 red pepper, deseeded and diced
1 tbsp mild chilli sauce
500g tomato passata
chopped fresh basil, to garnish

1 Cook the pasta in a large saucepan of boiling water along with the stock cube.
2 Meanwhile, heat a non-stick pan and dry-fry the onion and garlic for 4–5 minutes or until soft. Add the courgettes, red pepper, chilli sauce and passata and simmer gently until the vegetables are soft.
3 Drain the pasta, divide between warmed plates, top with the sauce and garnish with fresh basil.

Tomato and Asparagus Pasta ✔

Per serving 139 calories 1.2% fat
Serves 4 Prep time 10 mins Cook time 20 mins

180g pasta shapes
1 vegetable stock cube
1 small red onion, finely sliced
2 garlic cloves, crushed
250g fresh asparagus, chopped
400g tin chopped tomatoes
1 tsp vegetable stock powder
fresh basil and Parmesan, to garnish (optional)

1 Cook the pasta in a large saucepan of boiling water with
   the stock cube added.
2 Heat a non-stick pan and dry-fry the onion and garlic
   until soft. Add the asparagus, tomatoes and stock
   powder and simmer gently until the vegetables are soft.
3 Drain the pasta thoroughly and divide between warmed
   plates. Top with the sauce, then garnish with the basil
   and a little Parmesan if using.

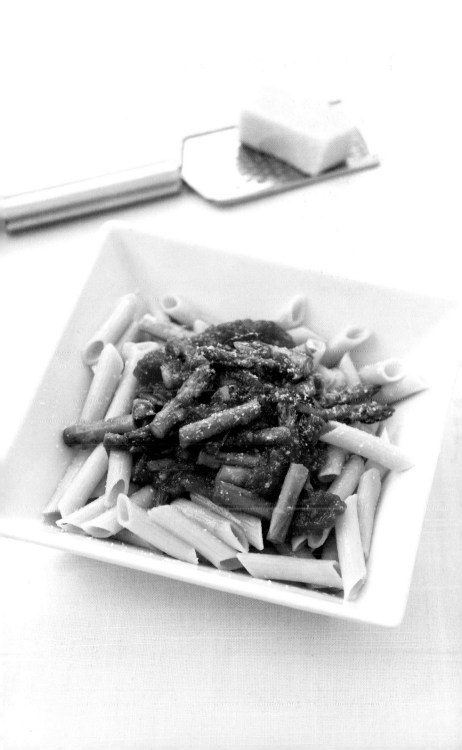

Spiced Squash Salad ✓

Per serving 153 calories 1.5% fat
Serves 4 Prep time 10 mins Cook time 15 mins

250g butternut squash, peeled and chopped
300ml (½ pint) boiling vegetable stock
1 tbsp harissa paste
200g couscous
juice of ½ lime
1 tbsp chopped fresh mint

1 Place the squash in a saucepan and add enough
   vegetable stock to just cover it. Simmer until soft, then
   drain, reserving the stock in a measuring jug. Make the
   stock up to 300ml with boiling water and mix in the
   harissa paste.
2 Meanwhile place the couscous in a large bowl, pour the
   hot stock over it and cover with a tea towel, allowing it to
   steam for 1–2 minutes.
3 Fluff up the couscous grains with 2 forks, stirring in the
   lime juice. Add the squash to the couscous along with
   the mint and mix well before serving.

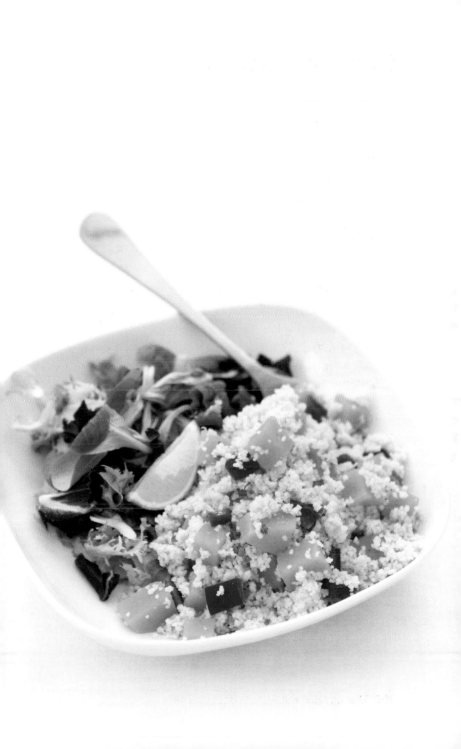

Goan Quorn Curry ⓥ

Per serving 118 calories 1.5% fat
Serves 4 Prep time 10 mins Cook time 25 mins

1 white onion, diced
2 garlic cloves, crushed
200g Quorn fillets, diced
2cm piece fresh ginger, peeled and finely chopped
1 red pepper, deseeded and diced
2 tsp Goan curry paste
200ml semi-skimmed milk
2 tbsp 2% fat Greek yogurt
salt and freshly ground black pepper, to taste
fresh coriander, to garnish

1 Heat a heavy-based, non-stick pan and dry-fry the onion
   and garlic until the onion is lightly browned.
2 Add the Quorn fillets and cook until sealed, seasoning
   with salt and black pepper. Stir in the chopped ginger,
   red pepper and Goan paste and continue to cook, mixing
   well, before adding the milk. Simmer gently for 20
   minutes until the sauce has reduced.
3 Just before serving, remove the pan from the heat and
   stir in the yogurt. Serve garnished with fresh coriander.

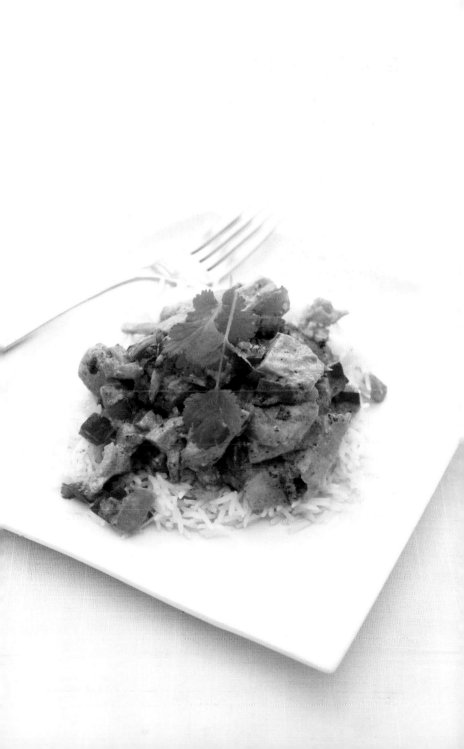

Quorn Rendang Curry ⊘

Per serving 161 calories 2.5% fat
Serves 4 Prep time 10 mins Cook time 20 mins

1 red onion, diced
2 garlic cloves, crushed
1 red pepper, deseeded and diced
350g Quorn pieces
1 tbsp rendang curry paste
150ml (¼ pint) pineapple juice
1 tsp vegetable stock powder
juice of ½ lime
2 tbsp 2% fat Greek yogurt
salt and freshly ground black pepper, to taste
chopped fresh coriander, to garnish

1 Heat a non-stick wok or frying pan and dry-fry the onion
   and garlic until soft. Add the diced pepper, Quorn pieces
   and curry paste and toss well, making sure the Quorn is
   heated through. Add the remaining ingredients, except
   the coriander, mix well and simmer for 10 minutes.
2 Transfer to serving plates and garnish with coriander.

Tomato, Basil and Cheese Tarts ✔

Per tart 210 calories 1.6% fat
Makes 2 Prep time 10 mins Cook time 25 mins

2 sheets filo pastry
4 spring onions, finely chopped
4 ripe tomatoes, skinned and chopped
3 tbsp tomato passata
50g low-fat mature cheese (max. 5% fat)
1 tbsp chopped fresh basil
low-cal spray oil, for cooking
freshly ground black pepper, to taste

1 Preheat the oven to 190°C, 375°F, Gas Mark 5.
2 Stack the filo pastry sheets on top of each other. Using
   scissors, cut the stack into 6 equal square sections, so
   that you end up with 12 individual squares.
3 Take 2 non-stick tartlet tins about 12cm in diameter. In
   each tin, layer 6 individual pastry squares, placing the
   squares at slight angles to each other and spraying with a
   mist of oil in between each layer. Bake the cases in the
   oven for 5 minutes until lightly browned.
4 In a mixing bowl, combine the spring onions, tomatoes,
   passata, cheese, basil and a little black pepper and
   spoon the mixture into the tart shells. Place on a non-
   stick baking tray and bake in the oven for 20–25
   minutes, until golden brown.
5 Allow to cool before removing from the tin.

Roasted Vegetable Sausages ⊘

Per serving 208 calories 3.2% fat
Serves 4 Prep time 10 mins Cook time 15–20 mins

300g pack vegetarian sausages
500g pack prepared roasting vegetables
1 red onion, cut into wedges
2 garlic cloves, sliced
2 tbsp thick balsamic vinegar
salt and freshly ground black pepper, to taste
low-cal oil spray, for frying
fresh parsley, to garnish

1 Preheat the oven to 200°C, 400°F, Gas Mark 6.
2 Place the sausages, roasting vegetables, onion wedges
   and garlic slices on a non-stick baking tray. Spray lightly
   with oil spray and season with salt and pepper, then cook
   in the oven for 15–20 minutes, until the sausages are
   brown and the vegetables are soft.
3 Remove from the oven and slice the sausages into
   chunks. Divide the sausage and vegetables between 4
   plates and drizzle with the balsamic vinegar.
4 Garnish with fresh parsley and serve.

Quick Mushroom Stir-Fry ⊘

Per serving 219 calories 1.3% fat
Serves 4 Prep time 10 mins Cook time 10 mins

2 red onions, finely sliced
2 garlic cloves, crushed
300g pack stir-fry vegetables
125g pack oyster mushrooms
300g thin rice noodles
150ml black bean sauce
1 tbsp mushroom ketchup
1 tbsp reduced-salt soy sauce
freshly ground black pepper, to taste

1 Heat a non-stick wok and dry-fry the onions and garlic
   for 2–3 minutes over a high heat, seasoning well with
   black pepper.
2 Add the stir-fry vegetables and oyster mushrooms to the
   pan and continue cooking for 1–2 minutes, then add the
   noodles and the remaining ingredients, tossing
   everything well together. Serve straight away.

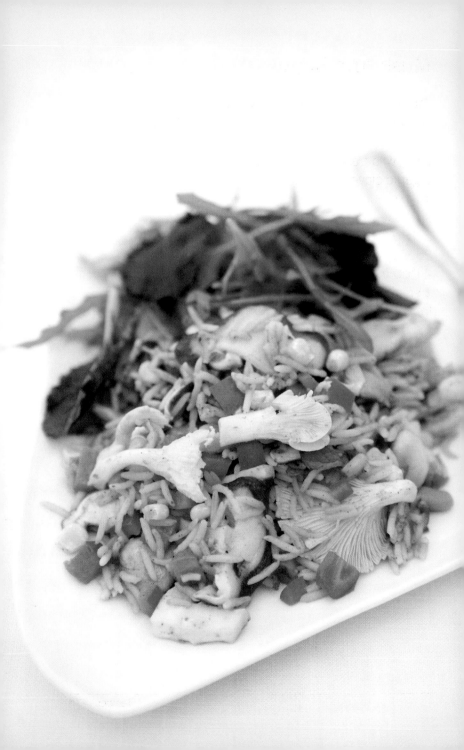

Mushroom Biryani ✅

Per serving 122 calories 1.5% fat
Serves 4 Prep time 5 mins Cook time 10 mins

250g wild fresh mushrooms, sliced
2 garlic cloves, crushed
1 tsp ground turmeric
1 red pepper, deseeded and diced
2 tbsp dry white wine
250g cooked rice
2 tbsp frozen sweetcorn
1 small red chilli, sliced
freshly ground black pepper, to taste
1 tbsp chopped fresh mint, to garnish

1 Heat a large non-stick frying pan and dry-fry the mushrooms and garlic until soft.
2 Add the turmeric and red pepper to the pan and cook for 1–2 minutes before adding the white wine. Stir in the rice, sweetcorn and chilli and cook until the sweetcorn is hot.
3 Transfer to serving plates and garnish with a little chopped mint.

Sweet Potato and Fruit Curry ✅

Per serving 274 calories 0.7% fat
Serves 4 Prep time 10 mins Cook time 20 mins

1 medium onion, chopped
1 garlic clove, crushed
2 green chillies, finely
   chopped
2.5cm piece fresh ginger,
   chopped
300ml (½ pint) vegetable
   stock
2 tsp garam masala
1 tsp ground coriander
1 tsp ground cumin

450g sweet potato, cut
   into chunks
225g green beans,
   trimmed
450g cauliflower florets
1 red pepper, deseeded
   and cut into chunks
300ml (½ pint) tomato
   passata
2 bananas
salt, to taste

1 Heat a large non-stick pan. Add the onion, garlic, chillies
   and ginger to the hot pan, cover with a lid and dry-fry for
   5 minutes over a gentle heat. Add a little vegetable stock
   if the mixture becomes too dry. When the onion is soft,
   stir in 3–4 tablespoons of the vegetable stock and
   sprinkle the spices into the pan. Cook for 1 minute,
   stirring continuously.
2 Add the sweet potato, beans, cauliflower and red pepper
   to the pan. Cook over a moderate heat for 2–3 minutes,
   stirring continuously. Pour in the remaining vegetable
   stock and the passata. Season to taste with salt, then
   cover the pan and cook gently for 10 minutes.
3 Peel and slice the bananas and add to the pan. Cook for
   a further 10 minutes or until the vegetables are tender.

Leek, Broccoli and Cauliflower Cheese ⓥ

Per serving 184 calories 1.7% fat
Serves 4 Prep time 15 mins Cook time 20 mins

200g fresh broccoli
200g fresh cauliflower
1 vegetable stock cube
4 leeks, chopped
500ml semi-skimmed milk
1 tsp vegetable stock powder
1 tbsp arrowroot
1 tsp English mustard powder
100g low-fat mature cheese (max. 5% fat), grated
freshly ground black pepper, to taste
1 tbsp chopped fresh chives, to garnish

1 Preheat the oven to 200°C, 400°F, Gas Mark 6.
2 Cut the broccoli and cauliflower into florets and put in a
   shallow pan of boiling water together with the stock cube.
   Add the leeks and then lightly cook the vegetables. Drain
   well and transfer to an ovenproof dish.
3 Pour the milk into the saucepan, add the stock powder
   and heat to near boiling. Mix the arrowroot with a little
   extra cold water and whisk into the hot milk along with
   the mustard powder and half the cheese. Simmer until
   the sauce has thickened, then pour the sauce over the
   vegetables in the ovenproof dish. Sprinkle the remaining
   cheese over the top and season with black pepper.
4 Bake in the oven for 20 minutes until brown on top.
   Serve garnished with the chives.

Watercress and Tomato Pasta ✓

Per serving 228 calories 0.6% fat
Serves 4 Prep time 5 mins Cook time 25 mins

180g pasta shapes,
1 vegetable stock cube
1 small red onion, finely diced
2 garlic cloves, crushed,
1 red pepper, deseeded and finely diced
500g pack tomato passata
100g fresh watercress
a little grated low-fat mature cheese (max. 5% fat),
    to garnish

1 Cook the pasta in a large saucepan of boiling water with
   the stock cube added.
2 Meanwhile, heat a non-stick pan and dry-fry the onion
   and garlic until soft. Add the red pepper and passata and
   simmer gently until the pepper is soft. Stir in the
   watercress.
3 Drain the pasta thoroughly and arrange on warmed
   plates. Pour the sauce over the pasta and garnish with a
   little grated low-fat cheese.

Spicy Mini Pizza ⓥ

Per serving 233 calories 2.1% fat
Serves 2 Prep time 5 mins Cook time 5 mins

1 small panini, approx. 80g
200g pouch Rosemary Conley Low-Fat Piri Piri Sauce
1 small red onion, sliced
1 beef tomato, sliced
20g low-fat mature cheese (max. 5% fat)
fresh basil leaves, to serve

1 Preheat the grill to high. Cut the panini in half and lightly
   toast on both sides.
2 Spread the bread with the piri piri sauce and top with
   onion, tomato and cheese. Return to the grill until golden
   brown. Serve garnished with fresh basil leaves.

Spicy Tagliatelle with Tomato and Chilli Sauce ⓥ

Per serving 246 calories 0.9% fat
Serves 2 Prep time 5 mins Cook time 20 mins

100g (dry weight) tagliatelle pasta
1 small vegetable stock cube
½ red pepper, finely chopped
1 small garlic clove, crushed
200g pouch Rosemary Conley Low-Fat Tomato
　and Chilli Sauce
1 tbsp chopped fresh basil, plus extra to garnish
salt and freshly ground black pepper, to taste
cherry tomatoes, to garnish

1 Cook the pasta in a large pan of boiling water containing the stock cube.
2 Meanwhile, heat a large non-stick frying pan and dry-fry the pepper and garlic until soft. Stir in the tomato and chilli sauce and bring to a gentle simmer, seasoning with salt and black pepper.
3 Stir in the basil and reduce the heat. Drain the pasta and divide between serving plates. Remove the sauce from the heat and spoon the sauce on top. Garnish with cherry tomatoes and fresh basil.

Desserts

Blueberry Chocolate Soufflés

Per serving 106 calories 1.6% fat
Serves 4 Prep time 10 mins Cook time 15 mins

200ml semi-skimmed milk
1 tbsp Green & Black's cocoa powder, sifted
1 tbsp cornflour
1 tbsp caster sugar
150g blueberries
2 egg whites

1 Preheat the oven to 200°C, 400°F, Gas Mark 6.
2 In a pan, heat most of the milk (reserving a couple of tablespoons) to near boiling, then whisk in the cocoa powder.
3 In a jug or bowl, mix the cornflour with the reserved milk until it forms a paste, then stir it into the cocoa powder mix. Simmer for a few minutes to allow the mixture to thicken, then remove from the heat and stir in the caster sugar and blueberries.
4 In a separate, clean bowl, whisk the egg whites until they form stiff peaks, then fold into the mixture. Pour into 4 ramekin dishes and bake in the oven for 15 minutes. Serve immediately as they will collapse as soon as they come out of the oven.

Chocolate Frozen Yogurt

Per serving 81 calories 0.6% fat
Serves 4 Prep time 10 minutes Freeze time overnight

500g 0% fat Greek yogurt
1 tsp xylitol sugar or other low-cal sweetener
3 tsp Green & Black's cocoa powder
4 tsp concentrated chocolate extract
4 mint leaves and a few red berries, to decorate

1 Put the yogurt in a mixing bowl and carefully fold in the
   sugar, cocoa powder and chocolate extract, taking care
   not to over-mix, until all the ingredients are combined.
   Pour into a freezer container and freeze until set, ideally
   overnight.
2 Decorate with a mint leaf and a few red berries on
   serving.

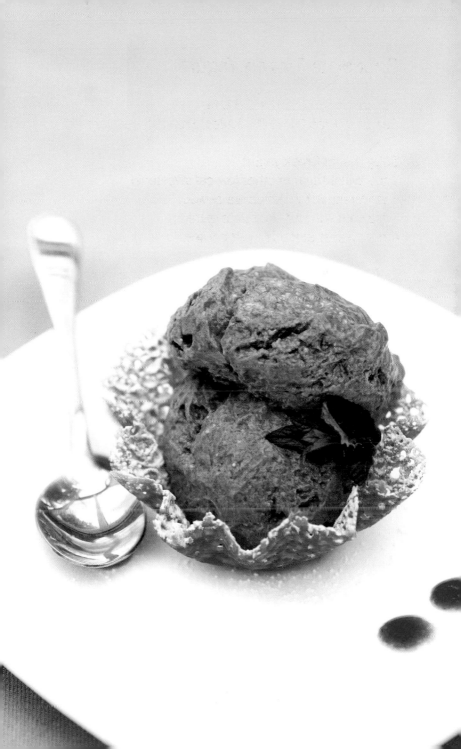

Lemon and Blueberry Pancakes

Per serving 115 calories 3.8% fat
Makes 6 Prep time 20 mins Cook time 10 mins

for the pancake batter
100g plain flour
1 egg
1 tbsp low-fat yogurt
1–2 tbsp skimmed milk
low-cal oil spray, for frying

for the filling
2 tbsp low-fat lemon curd
200g blueberries

to serve
a little caster sugar, to decorate
2 tbsp 0% fat Greek yogurt

1 To make the pancake batter, sift the flour into a mixing bowl, add the egg and yogurt and whisk together, adding sufficient milk to form a thick paste.
2 Heat a non-stick frying pan and spray lightly with oil spray. Cook the pancakes in batches. For each pancake, drop 1 tablespoon of the batter into the pan and cook for 1 minute, then flip it over and cook on the other side. Remove from the pan and keep warm while you make the remaining pancakes.
3 Spread the warm pancakes with the lemon curd and sprinkle with the blueberries. Roll up and sprinkle with a little caster sugar, then warm through in a low oven. Serve warm topped with a little 0% fat Greek yogurt.

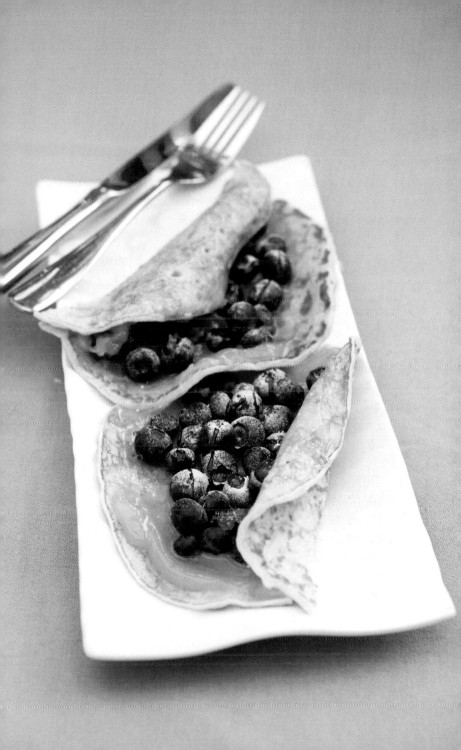

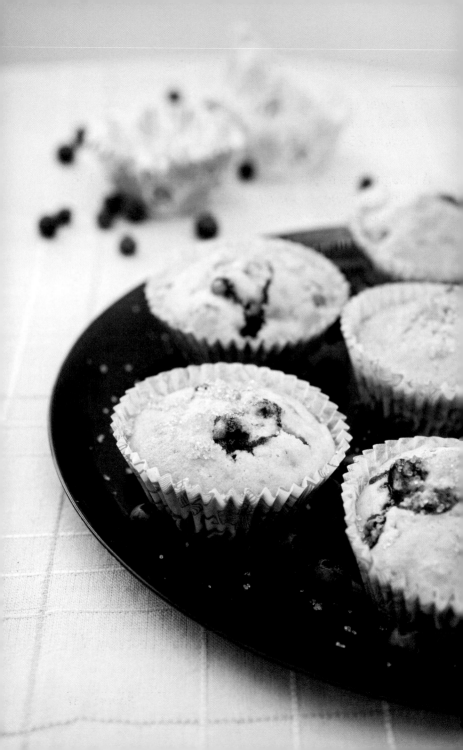

Blueberry and Lemon Muffins

Per muffin 198 calories 4.3% fat
Makes 6 muffins Prep time 10 mins
Cook time 20–25 mins

Although these muffins might seem high in calories, at 198 calories each, they are low in fat and have considerably fewer calories than their shop-bought equivalents.

85g low-fat spread
85g caster sugar
2 eggs, beaten
130g plain flour
1 tsp baking powder
zest and juice of 1 lemon
1 tbsp skimmed milk
100g fresh or frozen blueberries
1 tbsp demerara sugar

1 Preheat the oven to 150°C, 300°F, Gas Mark 2. Line a 6-muffin mould with muffin papers.
2 Cream together the low-fat spread and sugar in a large bowl, using a whisk. Gradually mix in the beaten eggs.
3 Sift in the flour and baking powder and add the lemon zest, mixing together with a wooden spoon to combine well. Mix in the skimmed milk and blueberries, then divide the mixture between the muffin papers.
4 Bake in the centre of the oven for 20–25 minutes until well risen and golden brown.
5 Mix together the lemon juice and sugar. Remove the muffins from the oven and, while still warm, drizzle with the lemon juice and sugar mixture.

Macaroons

Per macaroon 138 calories 0.6% fat
Makes 12 (sandwiched together) Prep time 10 mins
Cook time 30 mins

125g plain flour
200g icing sugar
3 egg whites
2 tbsp caster sugar
½ tsp cream of tartar
1 tsp almond flavouring
drop of food colouring (optional)

for the filling
2 tsp low-fat spread
2 tbsp icing sugar
1 tsp vanilla extract

1 Preheat the oven to 200°C, 400°F, Gas Mark 6. Line a non-stick baking tray with baking parchment.
2 Sift the flour and icing sugar into a bowl. In a separate, clean bowl, whisk the egg whites until stiff, then add the sugar a spoonful at a time while still whisking. Using a metal spoon, carefully fold in the flour, cream of tartar and almond flavouring, adding a drop of food colouring if desired.
3 Place the mixture in a piping bag and pipe 24 small walnut-sized dots onto the parchment-lined baking tray. Bake for 10 minutes. Remove from the oven and allow to cool before peeling off the paper.
4 Mix together the low-fat spread, icing sugar and vanilla extract. Spread half the macaroons with the mixture and top with the remaining macaroons.

Raspberry Traybake

Per serving 121 calories 4.2% fat
Serves 12 Prep time 10 mins Cook time 25 mins

3 sheets filo pastry
3 tbsp low-sugar raspberry jam
50g Lighter Than Light Flora
45g caster sugar, plus extra to decorate
2 eggs, beaten
60g self-raising flour
1 tsp almond flavouring

1 Preheat the oven to 150°C, 300°F, Gas Mark 2. Line a non-stick baking tray (about 16 x 25cm) with baking parchment. Layer the filo sheets over the baking parchment, spraying lightly with oil spray in between each sheet. Spread the jam over the pastry with a palette knife.
2 Using an electric whisk, cream together the low-fat spread and the 45g caster sugar. Whisk in the beaten eggs until combined, then stir in the flour and almond flavouring. Spread the mixture over the jam and bake in the oven for 25 minutes until golden brown. Sprinkle with a little more caster sugar before cutting into squares. Serve warm.

Ramekin Cheesecakes

Per serving 134 calories 4.7% fat
Makes 4 Prep time 15 mins Chill time overnight

1 vanilla pod
200g extra-light soft cheese
2 tbsp half-fat crème fraîche
2 tbsp low-sugar fruit jam
2 egg whites
12 amaretti biscuits
1 tbsp dry sherry
low-cal oil spray, for greasing
fresh fruit, to decorate

1 Lightly grease 4 ramekin dishes with oil spray, then line
   with clear food wrap, allowing it to hang over the sides of
   the dishes.
2 Split the vanilla pod in half with a small knife, scrape out
   the seeds into a mixing bowl and add the cheese and
   crème fraîche. Heat the jam in a small saucepan and stir
   into the mixture.
3 In a separate, clean bowl, whisk the whites and then fold
   into the cheese mixture. Spoon the mixture into the
   ramekins and press down.
4 Place the biscuits in a plastic food bag and crush with a
   rolling pin. Transfer to a small bowl and mix in the sherry.
   Press the biscuit topping over the cheesecakes, then
   cover and leave to chill in the fridge overnight. When
   ready to serve, turn out onto plates and decorate with
   fresh fruit.

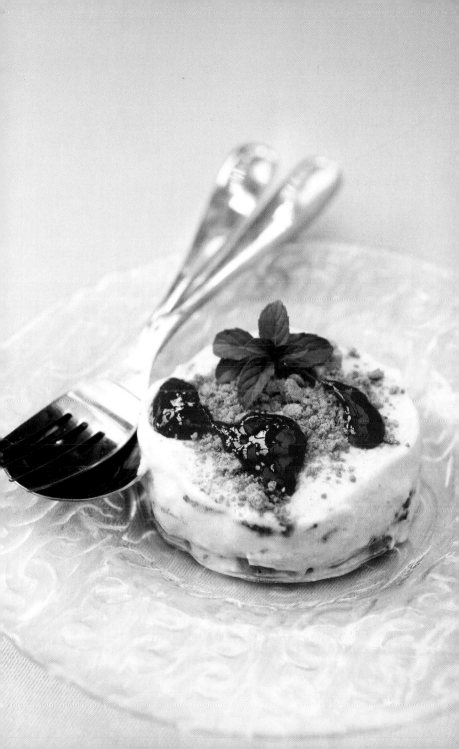

Chocolate Whoopie Cakes

Per cake 88 calories 7.6% fat
Serves 12 Prep time 15 mins Cook time 20 mins

These chocolate whoopie cakes make an ideal low-cal treat.

4 eggs
100g caster sugar
1 tsp boiling water
75g plain flour
30g Green and Black's
   cocoa powder
1 tsp vanilla extract

2 tsp Lighter Than Light Flora
2 tbsp icing sugar, plus
   extra for dusting
low-cal oil spray, for greasing
12 glacé cherries and
   2 tsp grated chocolate,
   to decorate

1 Preheat the oven to 180°C, 350°F, Gas Mark 4. Lightly grease a 12-hole silicone bun tray with a little oil spray.
2 Using an electric whisk, beat the eggs and sugar together on high speed for a few minutes. Add the boiling water and continue whisking until the mixture has more than doubled in volume and is thick and pale in colour.
3 Sift the flour and cocoa powder into a bowl then, using a metal spoon, carefully fold into the meringue mixture. Add the vanilla and continue mixing until fully combined. Pour into the bun tray, dividing the mixture evenly, and level the tops with a knife. Bake in the centre of the oven for 20 minutes until dry to the touch.
4 Turn the whoopies out onto a wire rack and allow to cool. In a bowl, mix together the low-fat spread and icing sugar to make a paste, then spoon into a piping bag and pipe on over each whoopie. Finish with a cherry on top. Just before serving, sprinkle with a little grated chocolate and dust with icing sugar.

Flapjacks

Per flapjack 84 calories 7% fat
Serves 12 Prep time 10 mins Cook time 25 mins

Although these flapjacks are 7% fat, they are allowed on my
FAB Diet because of the healthy oats they contain.

90g Lighter Than Light Flora
3 tbsp golden syrup
165g porridge oats

1 Preheat the oven to 180°C, 350°F, Gas Mark 4.
2 Heat the low-fat spread and golden syrup in a heavy-
   based saucepan until combined. Stir in the oats until
   coated. Pour into a non-stick baking tin (16 x 25cm)
   and level the top with the back of a metal spoon or
   palette knife.
3 Bake in the oven for 25 minutes or until golden brown.
   While still warm in the tin, cut into squares and then
   allow to cool completely before removing from the tin.
   Serve cold.

10
Move it!
Burn fat faster and get a FAB body shape

To maximise your weight loss on the FAB Diet, ideally aim to do some form of aerobic exercise every day. Every single extra step you take burns more calories, and yet most people go through the entire day without ever feeling out of breath. Doing any physical activity on a very regular basis at a level that increases your heart rate and causes you to breathe more deeply will help you burn extra calories as the body calls upon its fat stores to provide the fuel.

As well as burning fat and calories, aerobic exercise – also known as cardio work – increases the body's metabolic rate, not just during the activity itself but also for several hours afterwards through a process known as 'thermogenesis'. So even when you stop exercising, your body will keep burning lots of extra calories at a higher rate. How brilliant is that? Another bonus is that aerobic exercise helps your skin shrink as you slim. And the more you exercise, the slimmer you will become.

As you lose weight, doing regular physical activity will help to maximise the loss of body fat while preserving your muscle tissue, which will help maintain your metabolic rate and speed up your weight loss. Over time, exercise will boost your fitness, helping to control your blood pressure, raise the proportion of HDL (good) cholesterol in your bloodstream and reduce the risk of developing diabetes. By increasing the amount of exercise you do, alongside a healthy diet, you can gain the greatest health benefits.

Brisk walking, jogging, aerobic dancing, cycling and swimming are all excellent aerobic exercises that will burn fat and speed up your weight loss. There are many other forms of exercise that you may choose to undertake but I have set out a simple daily fitness challenge as part of the four-week plan, which could involve anything from walking up and down stairs consecutively or going for a 30-minute brisk walk. The recommendations for each day are progressive, so please make the effort to do them. By the end of the four weeks you'll find you can do significantly more than you could a month earlier. And do try my Five-Minute Core Workout in Chapter 11 – these three simple Pilates moves will streamline your waist and tone your tummy like you wouldn't believe. I used these exercises to improve my core strength when I was a contestant on ITV1's *Dancing On Ice* in 2012, and I still do them four or five times a week. Add them on to your daily fitness challenges, or if you're pushed for time and don't do anything else that day, then at least make sure you do this Pilates workout as it's a great all-round body toner and strengthener that will also help improve your posture and balance, and it takes just five minutes.

At the end of the first four weeks, if you're up for more of a challenge and want to get seriously fit, you can progress to the Advanced FAB Fitness Challenge – a six-week cardio and toning programme – in Chapter 12.

If you have a pedometer, wear it every day to check how active you are. Aim to achieve 10,000 steps a day, or at least 2,000 more steps than your usual number, as this will help you to lose your excess weight and also to maintain it once you have achieved a healthy weight.

Get a better body shape

If you want to have a great body shape, doing some toning or strength exercises three to five times a week will make your muscles firmer and stronger, which will improve your body shape and make you better equipped to carry out everyday tasks. Using resistance in the form of a resistance band or light handweights will make toning exercises more effective and enable you to see faster results. Start with 0.5kg weights or 500ml water bottles and then progress to 1kg weights or 1 litre water bottles.

Muscle tissue is energy-hungry and our muscles are our calorie-burning powerhouses. The stronger our muscles, the higher our metabolic rate and the more efficient our bodies will become at burning fat all the time, not just when we're exercising. Every time we move, we are using our muscles, so let's move more in our everyday life by using the stairs more, walking more and driving less.

Why toning exercises are good for you

- They make your muscles more dense and much firmer so the fat on top is less likely to hang loose!
- They give you a great shape, making you look leaner and slimmer.
- They turn you into a better fat-burner – toned muscles burn more calories even when you're not exercising.
- They make you stronger so that everyday tasks are easier.

Stretching

After an exercise session, it's good to stretch out the main muscles you've been using in order to prevent soreness later. On pages 317–321 you'll find the key stretches that are recommended after undertaking aerobic activity. It's worth learning them so you can do them after you've done a big hike or any other activity that challenges your leg muscles.

Do each stretch slowly and take care to get into the correct position, otherwise the stretch won't be effective in releasing the build-up of lactic acid that can cause aching muscles a day or two later. Hold each stretch in the extreme position for the count of 10 seconds and then release. You only need do each stretch once.

Break it down

Many people could increase their fitness just by adding a little more exercise to their daily routine, so if you can't manage 30 or 40 minutes at a time, break it down into five- or ten-minute slots. If you don't like formal exercise, find easy ways to incorporate more activity into your everyday life and then gradually increase the amount you do. Once you get into the habit of regular exercise, it will become second nature and you'll reap lifelong benefits.

Standing burns more calories than sitting. Realise that when you are sitting watching TV you are only burning around one calorie a minute. And what do we often do when we watch television? We eat! So not only are we hardly burning any calories, we are loading unnecessary extra calories into our body which means we have to work extra hard to burn those calories off!

If we get off the sofa and start moving more, we will increase our calorie output massively – possibly by 10 times as much depending on how active we are. If we walk, we'll increase our energy output from one calorie a minute when we were sitting down, to five calories a minute as we walk. If we jog or run, we could be burning 10 calories a minute. Doing aerobic exercise for 30 minutes could burn 300 calories, again depending on how energetic we are.

How to burn 100 calories

30 mins ballroom dancing

20 mins brisk walking

20 mins housework

15 mins jogging

15 mins swimming

10 mins high-impact aerobics

10 mins skipping

Easy ways to get more active

- Use a home exercise machine, such as a stationary bike or rowing machine – even if it's just for five minutes – or do a few sit-ups while watching your favourite TV soap or programme.
- Do a few squats or lunges while you're waiting for the kettle to boil.
- Walk up the stairs instead of taking the lift – it's a great fat-burner and bottom toner.
- At home make it a rule never to leave anything at the bottom of the stairs to take up later. Do it now.
- Get off the bus a stop earlier and walk the rest of the way.
- Go for a walk in your lunch break – even if it's only walking around the shops!

- Find an exercise buddy and arrange to meet up at the same time each week for a walk, jog, swim, bike ride, etc. You won't want to let your friend down and it's more fun exercising with others.
- Put extra vigour into your housework. Vacuuming is a great fat-burning exercise, so play your favourite music and turn your hoovering into an aerobic workout. It really works.
- Take the dog out for more walks and walk faster and further!
- Buy a skipping rope and skip for 2 minutes twice a day.

Remember, every bit of activity counts towards making you slimmer and fitter!

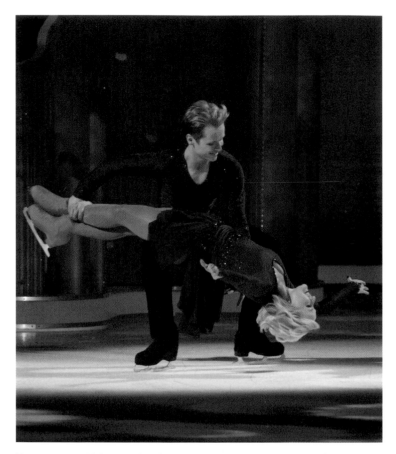

Rosemary and Mark performing the cantilever lift where core strength is essential. (KenMcKay / Rex Features)

11

The Five-Minute Core Workout

As soon as I received the news that I had been selected to appear on ITV1's *Dancing On Ice* in September 2011 I knew I needed to develop my core strength. I realised that if I was going to be lifted by my partner, be held in all kinds of weird and wonderful positions, I had to be able to hold my body together and not flop all over the place!

I was introduced to international professional ice skater Mark Hanretty on 7th November 2011. It was a memorable moment. I was asked to stand with my back to the rink and, only when instructed, to turn around. As I turned I saw this gorgeous, athletic, young man who was skating like a ballet dancer. My eyes filled up as it dawned on me that Mark was going to teach me to skate and that we were going to work together to turn me into something of a skater over the next few weeks and months, in the hope that we could stay in the competition for more than a week or two.

I had auditioned for *Dancing On Ice* three times before but been unsuccessful. I'd had a few lessons over the previous couple of years so that hopefully I'd at least be able to move forwards and backwards on the ice. As Mark and I started to skate together we developed a lovely partnership. And when Mark picked me up for our first 'lift', he said those magic words every woman wants to hear: 'You're so light!'

Mark didn't seem bothered that I was older than him, and we worked hard and well together to develop my skating skills – around three hours a day, six days a week. We also worked hard off the ice, practising my posture, leg positions and the lifts – which were always fun to do. That was when I realised that I needed to develop my core strength.

Mary Morris is the training consultant for Rosemary Conley Diet and Fitness Clubs, she writes for my magazine and has choreographed the last 18 of my fitness DVDs. Mary is also a great friend and the oracle of all things to do with exercise. More recently, she has qualified as a Pilates teacher and I knew that Pilates would be the answer to my core strength development. So it was to Mary that I turned for advice and training.

My request was simply: 'I know I will only do five minutes a day, but I promise I will do what you tell me every day.'

It wasn't long before my core strength was really tested. Included in the dance routine for our fourth skate on *Dancing On Ice* was the cantilever lift, where I was lifted onto Mark's bent knee with both of my legs outstretched and ankles crossed. Mark pressed down on my shins as I laid out flat with no support, hands above my head and only my stomach muscles to stop me dropping on to the ice. With my head only inches from the ice and Mark whizzing round in a sort of bent splits position, it was an interesting exercise! Then I had to pull my tummy muscles right in to lift myself up again, before Mark gently placed me back on my feet on the ice once more for us to continue.

And included here are the three core-strengthening exercises that Mary taught me. They were incredibly effective. I started off at the lower level and then progressed to the advanced versions. I still do them four or five times a week and they have toned up my waist and stomach like never before. The spare tyre has gone and my legs are more streamlined than ever – though if you want to have good legs and a toned bottom, take up ice skating. It works miracles! (If you would like to learn how to skate, why not join Mark and me at one of our Skate into Shape days, which we hold around the UK. Check out my website www.rosemaryconley.com/content/about-us/skate-into-shape.htm for details.)

I practise these three key Pilates exercises lying on my bathroom floor while waiting for my bath to run in the morning. I do them in addition to my other activities – this is a bonus workout! I really recommend you include them in your daily fitness routine. They will help you develop your core strength, streamline your body shape and improve your sense of balance. The 'Hundred' will strengthen your abdominal muscles – both the transversus abdominis muscle, which is the muscle that wraps around your middle like a corset, and also the obliques, or waist muscles, which lie at the sides of your trunk. In addition, the 'Torpedo' will work your hips and thighs, and the 'Dart' will strengthen the postural muscles in your spine. So you get a great all-round workout in just three moves!

The Hundred
Level one
Lie on your back with your feet off the floor, knees and feet together and knees bent at a 90-degree angle to your hips. Pull your shoulder blades down to stabilise your shoulders and reach both arms forward as you curl your head and shoulders off the floor, pulling your navel in towards your

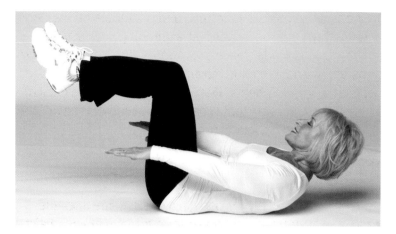

spine and keeping your chin off your chest. Now beat your arms up and down in tiny movements, breathing in for 5 beats and then out for 5 beats. Begin by counting up to 20 or 30 and gradually add more counts up to a maximum of 100. (Place a large rolled-up towel under your head if you want so you can rest your head down at any time.)

Level two
Lie on your back and start with knees bent as in Level One. Pull your navel in towards your spine and keep your chin off

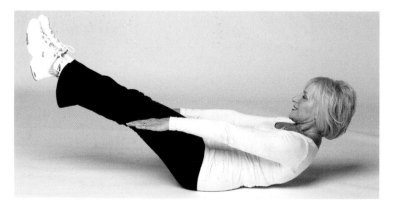

your chest as you curl your head and shoulders off the floor and reach your arms forward, straightening your legs fully so they form a 45-degree angle to your hips. Now beat your arms up and down in tiny movements, breathing in for 5 beats and out for 5 beats. Keep your head and trunk still at all times and on every 'out breath' try pulling your navel in a little more. Build up to a count of 100.

The Torpedo
Level one
Lie on your side with your body in a straight line from the hand over your head right down to your feet. Lift your waist away from the floor to stabilise your trunk. Breathe in as you lift the top leg to a 45-degree angle and hold it still Ⓐ, then breathe out as you lift the underneath leg to bring both legs together Ⓑ. Breathe in again, holding the legs still, then breathe out as you slowly lower the legs. Keep your waist lifted away from the floor and your navel pulled in

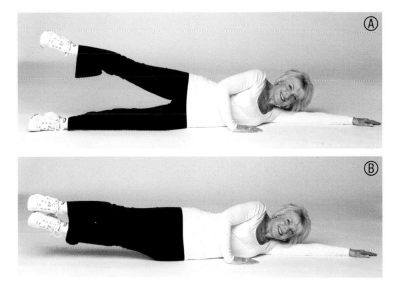

towards your spine throughout. Do 8 reps, then roll over and repeat on the other side.

Level two
Lie on your side with the body in a straight line as in Level One. Lift your waist away from the floor to bring your spine in line and stabilise your trunk. Now breathe in and lift both legs off the floor and then hold them still Ⓐ. Breathe out as you lift the top leg as high as you can without dropping the hips back Ⓑ, then breathe in and scissor the legs together, bringing the lower leg up and the top leg down. Breathe out again as you slowly lower both legs together. Do 10 reps, then roll over and repeat on the other side.

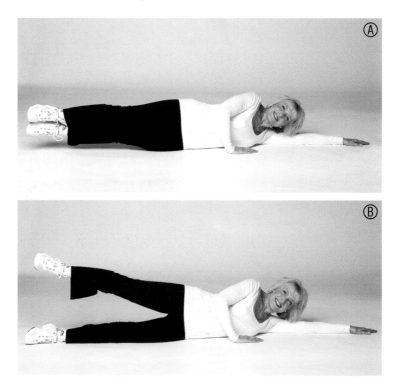

The Dart
Level one

Lie on your front with both arms bent in a diamond shape, elbows in line with your head, legs relaxed and hip-width apart Ⓐ. Breathe in and as you breathe out lift the back of your head towards the ceiling, but keep looking at the floor and keep your chin tucked in Ⓑ. Gently press your ribs into the floor to feel the muscles in the middle of your back working and pull your shoulders away from your ears. Hold still as you breathe in and then slowly lower your head as you breathe out. Do 6 reps.

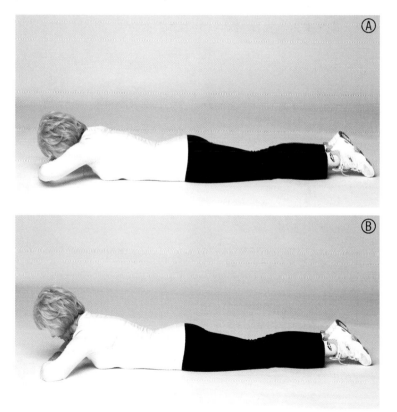

Level two

Lie on your front in the same position as Level One. Now breathe in and as you breathe out lift your head, pull your legs together Ⓐ, then take your arms out in front Ⓑ and sweep them round in one movement to bring them in line with your body Ⓒ, pulling your shoulder blades away from your ears. Hold still as you breathe in, and then as you breathe out slowly lower your head and return your arms to the start position. Do 8 reps.

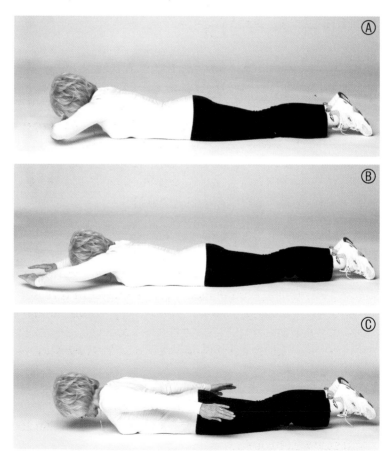

12
The Advanced FAB Fitness Challenge

Once you've completed the daily fitness routines in the four-week FAB Diet, if you're up for more of a challenge, then try this six-week Advanced FAB Fitness Challenge. It will continue to build your cardio strength as well as shape and tone your body – and get you really, really fit!
Try to persuade a friend to join you as it's a great way to boost your motivation. Find a fitness buddy with the same goals so you can support each other all the way.

How to follow the programme
The programme consists of a cardio challenge with a view to progressing your distance gradually. This is followed by a shaping and toning routine that will challenge both your upper body and core abdominal strength, giving you an all-round comprehensive programme. The programme is only a guide, so listen to your body and stop if you feel any pain.

Safety tips
- Make sure you feel warm before you start.
- Drink plenty of water before, during and after exercise so you stay well hydrated.

- Wear supportive trainers for the cardio challenge and try to mix the type of terrain you use, so that you walk or run on softer ground (such as grass) some of the time to reduce the stress on your joints.
- In the toning exercises, the number of reps is just a guide. Do enough to feel the muscle working hard without too much discomfort, and take a rest between sets.
- After each cardio session do the post-cardio stretches on pages 317–321 to stretch out the leg muscles, and after each toning session do the post-toning stretches to re-lengthen the muscles and prevent soreness later.

The FAB Cardio Challenge:
To walk/jog 5 kilometres (3.1 miles) in 45 minutes

Power walking
Power walking simply means adding power to your walk. Make a firm heel strike on each step and push off the front of the foot to propel you forward. There is no need to take bigger steps; you just need to make it more purposeful. Bending your elbows and holding them at waist height will automatically increase the power of your walking.

Gentle jogging
A good way to increase the intensity of your workout is to introduce short periods of gentle jogging. The definition of jogging is that at some point both feet are off the ground at the same time, which of course adds impact to your workout. As long as you do not have any major joint problems such as worn knees, hips or a recurring bad back, then a short period (1–2 minutes at a time) of gentle jogging will make you work harder and greatly increase the calorie-burning effect. Great news all round!

WEEK 1

Route: Flat

Warm-up walk for 5 minutes.

Power walk for a further 10 minutes.
(Optional: Add 3×1-minute of gentle jogging.)

Finish with a 2-minute cool-down walk,
followed by the post-cardio stretches.

Total workout time: 17 minutes

Number of sessions: 3

WEEK 2

Route: Flat

Warm-up walk for 5 minutes.

Power walk for a further 15 minutes.
(Optional: Add 3×2 minutes of gentle jogging.)

Finish with a 2-minute cool-down walk,
followed by the post-cardio stretches.

Total workout time: 22 minutes

Number of sessions: 3

WEEK 3

Route: Flat with some uphill

Warm-up walk for 5 minutes.

Power walk for a further 20 minutes.
(Optional: Add 3×3 minutes of gentle jogging.)

Finish with a 2-minute cool-down walk,
followed by the post-cardio stretches.

Total workout time: 27 minutes

Number of sessions: 3

Continued...

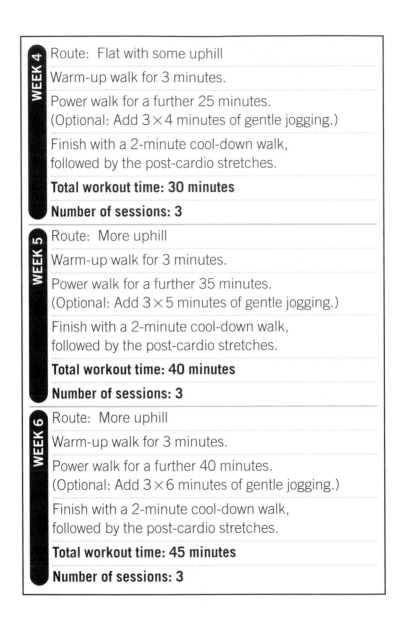

WEEK 4

Route: Flat with some uphill

Warm-up walk for 3 minutes.

Power walk for a further 25 minutes.
(Optional: Add 3×4 minutes of gentle jogging.)

Finish with a 2-minute cool-down walk,
followed by the post-cardio stretches.

Total workout time: 30 minutes

Number of sessions: 3

WEEK 5

Route: More uphill

Warm-up walk for 3 minutes.

Power walk for a further 35 minutes.
(Optional: Add 3×5 minutes of gentle jogging.)

Finish with a 2-minute cool-down walk,
followed by the post-cardio stretches.

Total workout time: 40 minutes

Number of sessions: 3

WEEK 6

Route: More uphill

Warm-up walk for 3 minutes.

Power walk for a further 40 minutes.
(Optional: Add 3×6 minutes of gentle jogging.)

Finish with a 2-minute cool-down walk,
followed by the post-cardio stretches.

Total workout time: 45 minutes

Number of sessions: 3

The FAB Shape and Tone Programme

This short but very effective shape and tone programme has only five exercises. That means you can complete it in just five minutes! The cardio programme on pages 310–312 is a great workout for all your leg muscles, so by adding these quick and simple toning exercises to your fitness regime you get an all-over body workout, leaving you beautifully firm and toned.

1. Shoulder shaper

Stand with feet apart and hold 2 × 1kg handweights (or 2 × 1-litre water bottles) at your sides.

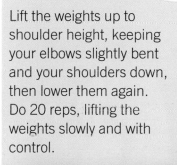

Lift the weights up to shoulder height, keeping your elbows slightly bent and your shoulders down, then lower them again. Do 20 reps, lifting the weights slowly and with control.

2. Waist trimmer

Stand tall with feet wider than shoulder-width and hold a 1kg handweight (or a 1-litre water bottle) with both hands. Pull your tummy in tight and lift the weight to head height Ⓐ. Now twist your trunk to one side and bend your knees as you lower the weight down to the outside of the opposite thigh Ⓑ. It's very important that you keep your knees in line with your feet. Lift the weight up again, then repeat to the other side. Do 20 slow reps, alternating sides.

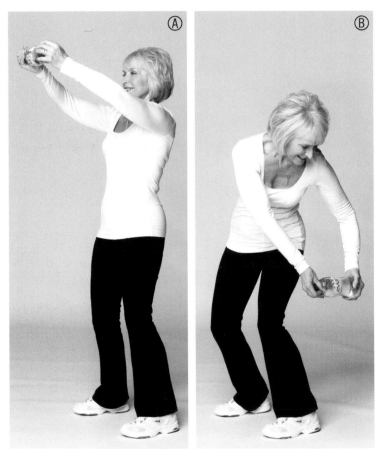

3. Chest and underarm firmer

Get down on your hands and knees, with wrists directly under your shoulders, knees under your hips (or slightly further back if you want to make it harder) and your tummy pulled in Ⓐ. As you breathe in bend your elbows outwards and lower your forehead just in front of your fingers Ⓑ. Breathe out as you push back up again without locking the elbows out at the top. Do 20 slow reps.

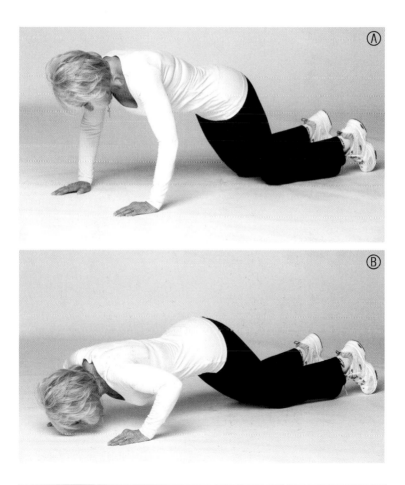

4. Tummy trimmer

Lie on your back with knees bent and feet hip-width apart, with a handweight or water bottle in one hand and holding it above your chest. Use the other hand to support your head. Breathe in and as you breathe out, lift your head and shoulders off the floor, pulling your tummy in and keeping your chin off your chest, then lower again. Do 20 reps, keeping them slow and controlled.

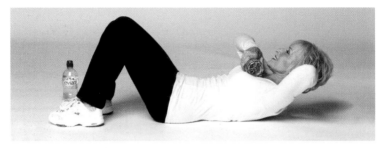

5. Half plank tummy flattener

Start by lying on your front with tummy pulled in tightly. Breathe in and as you breathe out, pull up onto your knees and elbows, with your hips in line with your head (check in a mirror if possible). Hold for 30 seconds, breathing normally and holding your tummy in throughout. Repeat.

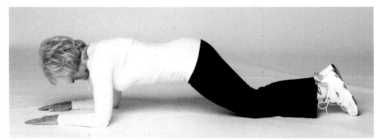

Remember to do the post-toning stretches on pages 322–323 at the end of each session.

Post-Cardio Stretches

1. Calf stretch

Take one leg back and bend the front knee, keeping the back leg straight. Check that both feet face straight ahead, then press the back heel down into the floor to increase the stretch in the calf of the back leg. Hold for 10 seconds, then do stretch 2 (lower calf stretch) before changing legs.

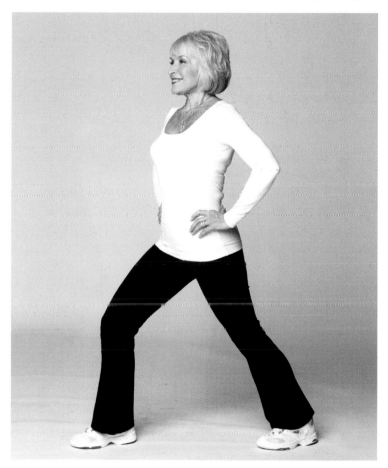

2. Lower calf stretch

Bring the back leg in half a step and bend both knees to feel a stretch in the lower calf of the back leg. Make sure both feet are facing straight ahead. Hold your body upright to increase the effect. Hold for 10 seconds, then repeat stretches 1 and 2 on the other leg.

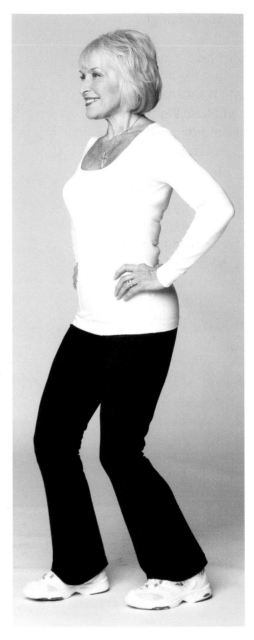

3. Front of thigh stretch

Take hold of one leg around the ankle with the same-side hand (use the back of a sturdy chair, or a sturdy fence or tree, for support if needed). Stand tall with tummy in and bring your knees in line, pressing the hip of the raised leg forward slightly. Hold for 10 seconds, then change legs and repeat.

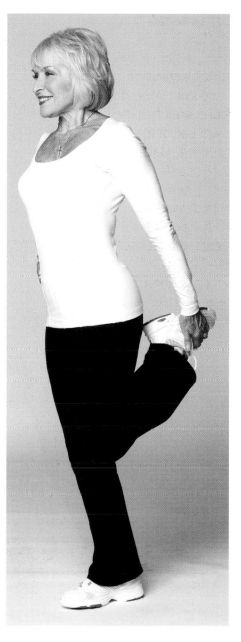

4. Back of thigh stretch

Place one foot in front of the other and lean forwards from the hip, keeping your back straight and resting your hands on your thighs, to feel a stretch at the back of the straight leg. Hold for 10 seconds, then rest and repeat on the other leg.

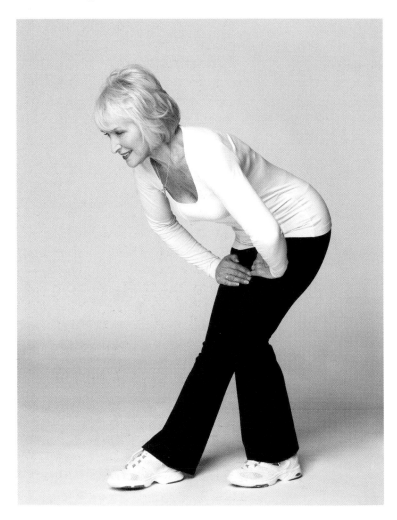

5. Inner thigh stretch

Stand with feet wider than shoulder-width apart and bend your right knee in line with the ankle. Turn your left foot to face forward and widen your stance to feel a stretch on the inner thigh of the left leg. Hold for 10 seconds, then change legs and repeat.

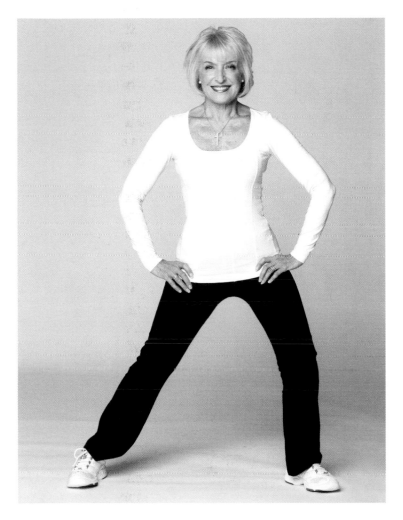

Post-Toning Stretches

6. Tummy stretch

Lie on your front with both arms out at your sides and your elbows bent. Now prop yourself up on your elbows and pull your chin up slightly to feel a stretch down the front of your trunk. Hold for 10 seconds, then slowly release.

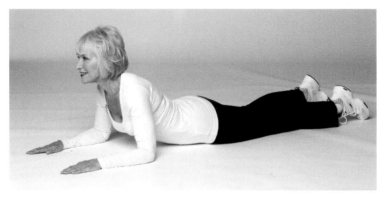

7. Chest stretch

Sit upright and place both hands behind you on the floor. Pull your shoulder blades together and then pull your shoulders down to feel a stretch across the front of your chest. Hold for 10 seconds, then slowly release.

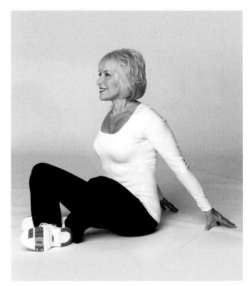

8. Underarm stretch

Sit upright with legs in a comfortable position and place your left hand at the back of your left shoulder. Use your right hand to gently press on the underarm to take the left hand further down your back, so that you feel a stretch in the left underarm. Keep your head up and in line with your spine. Hold for 10 seconds, then change arms and repeat.

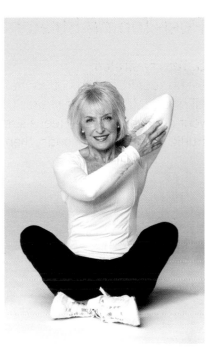

9. Shoulder stretch

Sitting upright, bring one arm across the front of your chest. Using your other hand, press the upper arm further across to feel a stretch in your shoulder. Hold for 10 seconds, then change sides and repeat.

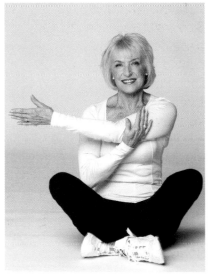

13
Staying slim: your FAB maintenance plan

Losing weight is a real learning curve. It can be a real eye-opener discovering which foods are high in fat and calories, and then there's the challenge of learning how to cook low fat and the discipline of making time to exercise. As you start to feel healthier and fitter, it's a wonderful feeling when you find you don't get out of breath so quickly and you feel your clothes are getting looser. Then there's the excitement of reaching your ultimate goal. Maybe you can't quite believe you've done it? All those weeks of hard work have paid off and now you're lapping up the compliments from family and friends. But what happens next? How do you keep the weight off?

Losing your excess pounds is a journey of discovery, but maintaining your new weight into the future can be more of a challenge. To avoid regaining weight, it's important to stick with your low-fat eating habits. Just as you can wean yourself away from the taste of high-fat foods, it's easy to retrain yourself back into your old, bad habits but if you do, you'll regret it. That doesn't mean you can't ever have a cream cake or a Big Mac. Of course you can – but only occasionally and see it as a treat and an exception rather than the rule.

I suggest you increase your calories by 200 a day, to see if you are able to keep your weight constant. If you find the weight starts to creep back on, cut down again. If at any time you overindulge, for instance on holiday, return to the Kick-Start Booster Diet for a few days. However, unless your BMR determines that 1200 calories is the correct number for your daily needs, don't stick to it long term, otherwise your willpower will break and you'll find yourself eating anything and everything!

If you're aged 60 or over, you will not be able to have more than about 1500 calories a day without putting on weight, unless you do a lot of exercise. Hopefully, you'll fall into a routine that allows you to eat enough and stay slim without feeling that you are dieting. I've managed to maintain my weight for a long time now. If I find I gain a little, I just cut back for a few days until I get back to my normal size. I hardly ever weigh myself at all and mostly go from the fit of my clothes.

Try not to obsess about your weight, and avoid stepping on the scales each day. Scales can motivate and de-motivate. If you've lost weight you might be tempted to eat more 'because you are in credit'. And if you've gained a pound you can go into panic mode and find yourself stressed and then immediately reach for your 'weakest-link' food such as biscuits, chocolate, or crisps. So try to relax and gradually you will build your self-confidence in controlling your eating.

To help keep your weight down, keep exercising regularly – aim to do 30 minutes of aerobic activity three to five times a week at a level that makes you mildly breathless and warm. Surveys of people who have lost weight and kept it off repeatedly show they have become regular exercisers – whether it's walking or cycling to work, joining a sports club, attending an exercise class or going to the gym. The fact is, without regular exercise you will need to consciously limit your appetite to avoid gaining weight.

On the other hand, there's growing evidence that regular exercise can help your body to control its food intake better and adjust your appetite naturally to meet your energy needs, so that you avoid regaining weight.

Enjoy the benefits of being fit and slim. Enjoy buying new clothes, enjoy running around with your children, and enjoy the compliments.

10 tips to help you keep your weight on track

1 Stick to eating three meals a day and don't skip any of them.
2 Continue to eat low fat and preparing and cooking food the low-fat way.
3 Stay active – aim for 30 minutes of aerobic exercise on three to five days a week.
4 Set yourself some new goals. Why not train to enter the Race For Life or even a half-marathon and raise money for your favourite charity? Finding a new physical challenge will encourage you to keep exercising, which will help you stay slim.
5 Take an 'after' photograph of yourself. Keep this photo handy, together with your 'before' picture, to remind yourself of how far you have come.
6 Take all your 'big' clothes to the charity shop – except for your very largest garment, which you should keep as a memento of how far you have come.

7 Make a conscious effort NOT to slip back into your old eating habits, like buying a bar of chocolate or bag of crisps every morning on your way to work.

8 Go easy on the alcohol. Enjoy a drink but try to limit yourself to two a day max. Avoid binge drinking. Apart from the effects on your health, having too much alcohol will delay the burning of body fat. The reason for this is that the body sees alcohol as a toxin so it gets rid of the alcohol calories first. This means any extra calories from food will be stored as fat.

9 You're not actually 'dieting' now, so if it's someone's birthday and it's cream cakes all round, feel free to have one. Enjoy it and appreciate it as a treat.

10 Don't step on the scales every day. You'll know if you've gained or lost weight from the way your clothes fit. If your clothes start to feel tight, return to the Kick-Start Booster Diet for a few days and do a bit more activity.

Most of all, give yourself a big pat on the back. You are slimmer, fitter and healthier now and you've worked hard to get that way. Remember, nothing tastes as good as being slim feels!

SLIMFILE

Naomi Baker

Age 39

Height 5ft 4in (1.63m)

Top weight 13st 4lb 4oz (84kg)

Now weighs 10st 7lb (67kg)

Total weight lost 2st 11lb 4oz (17kg)

Total inch loss 46in (117cm)

Dress size was 18/20 **now** 10

BMI was 32 **now** 25.2

INCH LOSS

Bust was 40in (102cm)
now 33in (84cm)

Waist was 35in (88.9cm)
now 28in (71cm)

Hips were 40in (102cm)
now 33in (84cm)

Widest part was 44in (110cm)
now 36in (91cm)

Left thigh was 25in (63cm)
now 20in (51cm)

Right thigh was 25in (63cm)
now 20in (51cm)

Left knee was 18in (46cm)
now 14½in (37cm)

Right knee was 18in (46cm)
now 14½in (37cm)

14
Naomi's weight-loss blog

After giving up work to start a family, Naomi Baker, 39, gained over 3st (19kg). She didn't want to be fat and forty so she joined rosemaryconleyonline.com, our online slimming club, and lost 2st 11lb 4oz (17kg) in 26 weeks. Here's her blog about her weight-loss journey.

My weight-loss journey: how it all started

I've been on some diet or other since my teenage years – although looking back at photos, I can see that half the time I didn't really need to lose weight.

From around the age of 22 until my early 30s, I worked hard – and partied harder! As an area supervisor responsible for 10 hair and beauty salons in the south of England, located between Plymouth and Milton Keynes, I spent many hours a week in my car and living in hotel rooms. My nights were spent socialising and trying to fill the void of not being at home, and this is when I began to put on weight in earnest.

In 2005 I went to work for a luxury cruise line, travelled the world and scored myself a wonderful husband. We had our first son in 2008. During my pregnancy I gained 40lb and struggled to lose it afterwards. We were living in Cyprus at the time and I bought a copy of Rosemary Conley's *Gi Hip and Thigh Diet* book online. I followed it as well as I could, but couldn't always get hold of the ingredients needed for certain recipes. I also walked up and down the seafront every day. I lost around 17lb and felt much better. I was still overweight though, with a BMI of 32. Shortly after this I suffered two miscarriages and began to comfort-eat to drown my sorrows.

In November 2010, I discovered I was pregnant again, with my now youngest son. Everything went really well and he was born in August 2011.

When I'm pregnant, I become 'Britain's Best Baker' and start baking, cakes, cookies, quiches… I give most of them away to friends but have been known to eat a few myself – for the purposes of quality control, of course! During my second pregnancy I gained around 50lb, which was the heaviest I'd ever been.

At the end of January 2012 when my youngest son was six months old, I decided to tackle my weight problem. This time I felt I needed the support and encouragement of a class – and I only wanted to do Rosemary Conley. It's the only plan I know that offers exercise as well as a weigh-in. Unfortunately, I couldn't get to a class as I don't have a car and my husband's shifts don't allow me to plan things on a weekly basis.

My sister, Rachel Baker – who's a Rosemary Conley Diet and Fitness Club franchisee in Devon – suggested I try rosemaryconleyonline.com and put me in touch with another franchisee, Lindsey Peters, in Hertfordshire. Lindsey was really helpful and agreed to give me support each week, alongside my sister.

After speaking with the online team I decided to give it a go. I had a two-week free trial and I absolutely loved it. It felt so good to be back in control of my life when everything else around me was chaos!

I helped my sister set up her franchise Facebook page when she started her diet and fitness classes and also offered to do a weekly blog so that I would be accountable to her members and, hopefully, that would keep me on track. It was a huge success and she now includes my blogs in her weekly newsletter. I've received many comments and support from her members. I'm very honest about how my week has gone – good or bad – and the readers seem to like it.

My sister forwarded my blogs to Rosemary and I was completely blown away when Rosemary called me at home one day and asked if she could include them in her new book. I feel totally honoured and couldn't write about something I didn't wholeheartedly believe in. This FAB Diet is amazing and I hope you enjoy it too.

Blog 1

This is my first blog entry on the Rosemary Conley path to weight loss.

In my 20s, I used to sit nicely around 9½ to 10½st.
In my 30s, that crept up to 11st, then 12st.
Now at age 38 and 11 months, and two children later, I weigh 13st 4lb 4oz. Not bad for all of 5ft 4in. During my last pregnancy I went up to 15st 11lb and looked like a Weeble! In the last six months I've lost some weight on my own but have come to a standstill.
Something has to change and soon. I am fast approaching my 'naughty forties' and do not want to be the weight I am now!

I am only on Day 3 so far and feel so much better and in CONTROL.

After clearing my cupboards of foods I knew were not going to be helpful, I made a shopping list and filled the cupboards with yummy foods for all the family. The one thing I've noticed already from looking at my new food diary is I don't drink ENOUGH WATER.

So this is it, no looking back or making excuses, I want to find the real me and not be tired any more or out of energy. My boys need a mummy who can run about with them. Watch this space…

Blog 2

So Week 1 is in the bag. I couldn't sleep all night on Tuesday as I was thinking about my weigh-in (and partly because baby Leo cried for two hours). I was excited but nervous.

I knew what I had eaten all week and felt sure I'd done a great job compared to previous weeks and months.

On Sunday I was faced with a very posh meal out and chose salmon and spinach from the menu, drank water but had NO DESSERT. Usually, I check out the dessert first so I can plan my main course around it. I was so proud of myself.

I hope I can keep making great choices, but if I do slip up, I'll try not to beat myself up and just get back on track.

It felt great to be in control of what was going into my body and I found that writing down every food item and drink showed me where I was flaking during the day and craving sugar fixes. I did crumble a little on one day – after a stressful day with the boys and little sleep, I wanted CHOCOLATE. I remembered reading about those Pink 'n' White wafers in the Rosemary Conley magazine, so I went to get some of those. Over the day, I ate all six (whoops!) but it could have been a lot worse – like a whole pack of digestive chocolate biscuits.

I also took my measurements and saw for myself where the inches had to go:

Boobs: 43in
Waist: 35in
Hips: 42in
Widest part: 44.5in

I am an hourglass with a few too many curves.

The anticipation rose on weigh-in day and I would have jumped out of bed, if I could but my back gave up on me during the week (another good reason to lose those unwanted lbs).

Today the scales said 12st 13lb 4oz. A whole 5lb off. Yippee! My hubby, who is 'technically' not on the plan, has lost a whopping 7lb.

We are aiming to lose about 40lb each, so we are well on our way and I'm sure our bed is going to be so grateful to have less weight on it.

Blog 3

Can't believe that two weeks have passed already and I still love every moment. I've been in various situations with friends and groups where biscuits and such like are free-flowing and I have not faltered! That does not mean I haven't eaten sweet things, I've been trying hard to make good choices.

Wednesday for me is weigh-in day and, just like last week, I was very excited!

The scales said 12st 10lb 8oz! That is another 2lb 12oz

gone and I got my first certificate online. Whoop whoop, over 7lb gone! Goodbye, not going to miss you! My body fat percentage also dropped by 1% and my BMI has gone from 32 to 31.something. Then for the tape measure, I'm sure I need markers painted on my body!

Boobs have lost 1in so far, waist 1in and another 4in from various other bits! Not bad for 16 days of enjoyment. Next was hubby Alex's turn. He too dropped another 2.7lb (total 9.7lb). He'd got all despondent, thinking he had gained weight. MEN! He too, has lost a few inches.

One thing that's really helping me is doing my shopping online. As we don't have a car, it's the only way I can keep my sanity! I prepare all my meals using the FAB weekly menu. The thing I love about the diet is you can swap one meal for another if there's something you don't like. I find this helps me stick to my shopping list because I don't buy things I don't need. Plus, there are no impulse-buy till displays loaded with chocolate!

My other discovery of the week – HOUSEWORK! I've not been able to exercise how I'd like to because of some back issues. I found a section on rosemaryconleyonline where I could enter everything I do on a daily basis – washing up, putting away dishes, making beds, cooking dinner… you get the picture. To my surprise, I burn nearly 700 calories doing my housekeeping bits every day. I've always loved cleaning (freak, I know) but now I *really* love it. I'm also going up and down the stairs as much as possible!

Blog 4

MY NAME IS NAOMI AND I AM AN EMOTIONAL EATER. I eat when I am happy, I eat when I am sad, I eat when I am anxious, I eat when I am tired, you name it, I eat it. This past week, I've been bombarded with all kinds of emotions from sleep deprivation from my early rising toddler and my teething, constipated baby to pure grief and disbelief at a friend's tragic news. All of these events would normally throw me into a spiral of comfort eating and hating myself, feeling like a failure, but the only difference this week is that I felt a little more in control of my actions. As I'd lost some weight already I had my 'good head' and was battling the 'devil's head' constantly. Good overcame bad most of the time.

It wasn't easy, though. I felt like I was becoming schizophrenic as the week went on! But all of these events did do one thing for me, which was to question why exactly did I want to be following the Rosemary Conley programme? I have messed about with so many diets before and, looking back over photos, I realise that most of those times I didn't need to be on a diet. Low self-esteem drove me there.

Of all my previous dieting attempts I did really well for the first four to five weeks and then after that I lost faith or got bored and started making excuses about why I had suddenly started to chomp my way through the bakery shelf in the supermarket again. I was cheating myself. I really do need to lose weight now, though. I am not in the obese end of the BMI scale but I am in the top end of the overweight scale, and the difference now is that I have a family that I want to be around for so I can set an example to my boys and give them the skills they need to make healthy choices. Hopefully, they will be able to cook an amazing meal for their partners in the future (and do the washing-up after).

The thing I love about Rosemary's FAB plan is that many of the meals are made from fresh (even her Solo Slim® ready meals are made from fresh ingredients) and most don't take more than 30 minutes. I can prepare one meal for the whole family and make the calorie value higher for my children by adding full-fat ingredients such as cheese.

I do hope I am now on my path for life and can learn to manage my 'emotional eating' habits. Maybe my good and bad angels can fight it out among themselves.

So, how did hubby and I do this week?

I am totally astonished as I have lost another 3lb 4oz and hubby almost 3lb. I've shed 11lb in total now and Alex 12lb. We are really beginning to feel the difference and are very excited about things to come.

Blog 5

In my quest to find more ways to burn calories, other than the obvious blood, sweat and tears methods, I came across a subcategory in the exercise listings on Rosemary Conley online.

I wasn't sure I had read it right at first, but there it was in black and white…

SEXUAL ACTIVITY! I almost choked on my decaf Earl Grey tea.

Ooh, let's take a peek at this, I thought to myself. Under further investigation, I discovered there were three ratings of sexual activity:

1) Active, vigorous effort.
2) General, moderate effort
3) Passive, light effort, kissing, hugging.

Now, I am sure some of you can relate to this. When Alex and I were in the process of baby making, I could say we easily fitted in to Category 1, like hurricane season, fast and furious. But that was more than 17 months ago.

Another baby later, and with Alex working 12 to 13-hour shifts as a chef and me as chief honcho in the house, cleaning clothes, dishes, noses, nappies, cooking, shopping blah blah blah… we might pass for Category 3! There's also the privacy issue now – with a toddler in the house, there's no time apart from the middle of the night when you can have 'love' time and that time is now for precious sleep, always conscious that Baby No. 2 might wake at any moment! My husband would love to be back in Category 1 and I am sure that day will come soon but for now, it is what it is.

So, out of interest I put in 10 minutes of Category 3, just to see how it might affect my efforts for weight loss – and it burnt all of 10 calories! I was shocked to see that 10 minutes of Category 1 burnt only 16 calories, so why should I bother to make that extra effort?

That got me to thinking about all the other 'users' online. Do they use this categorisation in their exercise sections? Surely the people at head office read this info to keep track of dieters' progress. Would people really admit to five to ten minutes of activity? Is that the norm? For my poor husband, 10 minutes with me is actually a great achievement right now. I've decided I am going to use this section only when I can hold my head up high and say that we had 60 minutes of vigorous effort, with no injuries occurring and no alcohol was involved! That said, it would still only burn 93 calories but it would be a highly enjoyable exercise session for all involved. At that point, I know I will be at target, wearing lovely matching underwear that's not just reserved for holidays and I'll get undressed with the lights on. Unlike now, wearing my unattractive nursing bras and old tatty knickers that have seen better days and will be recycled into cleaning rags! So for now, anything south of my belly button is remaining sacred ground, reserved for birthdays, anniversaries and Christmas, which reminds me, I still owe my hubby for his January birthday.

So the results for this week are (drum roll!)…

I lost ANOTHER 3lb! Hubby lost 2lb, making a total of 14lb each in four weeks. Our eldest son weighs 33lb, so another 5lb and we'll have shed a whole Ethan!

Blog 6

This week I was going to write about my new best friends but that was before various viruses invaded my house, my kids and my life and turned it upside down. This past week has been a tough one and, honestly, if I had not been housebound, I would have eaten my body weight in chocolate!

It all started at the weekend, Ethan was looking a little off colour and then BOOM, Monday morning he had a raging fever! No preschool and a tired mummy are not a great mix. Plus baby Leo had decided on Sunday night to start exercising his vocal cords every night, from around midnight until 4am. So basically my week has been housebound, with cabin fever, on duty 24 hours a day and hubby only had one day off, half of which he spent in bed with the worst case of man flu ever. Chills, sweats, fever, headache…

So, thank the Lord that I've planned my week's meals ahead, got my shopping online and that my dear friends did not respond to my desperate pleas on my Facebook page every day for CHOCOLATE! They are fully aware of my goals and want to support me. Some did offer to give in but my conscience got the better of me and I muttered a few gritted 'No thank yous'.

On weigh-in day, I did not feel confident at all, as the only exercise I had done all week was running around the house answering the needs of my boys. So I was really surprised to have lost another 2lb 2oz. It was the highlight of my week!

Hubby lost another 4lb!

In total I have lost 16lb 2oz and hubby has lost 18lb in 37 days! We are both really noticing it and getting compliments (when not housebound). My stats so far are:

16.75in lost
3.12in off my waist
BMI down to 30.14 from 32

I might get a few haters now, but I swear I've lost some cellulite from my hips and thighs – I think it's melting away! Thinking about my weight loss, I worked out that in the past 37 days I have consumed 56,000 calories less. It takes 3500 calories less to lose 1lb. What the hell was I eating before? I must have been eating so much of the wrong food, it's really scary.

Blog 7

I can't believe this is my seventh blog already. The weeks are flying by and the lbs are flying away. Last week's blog was all about my family's illnesses and I'm afraid it didn't get much better. I finally got struck down on Sunday by the deadly virus and spent most of the day in bed feeling sorry for myself. Even so, I think it would still have been a tough week anyway. Six weeks in, I'm getting comfortable with the RC way of eating and preparing food and I can feel some bad habits creeping back in. Making sandwiches for my son and nibbling on the crusts instead of chucking them out for the birds, thinking about chocolate all day long and needing some comfort foods. Week 6 for me was DANGER week and I don't think I would have got through it had it not been for two NEW BEST FRIENDS that have come into my life. These new friends have become staples in my everyday life and I crave them from the moment I wake up. My friends and lifesavers are:

1) My pedometer.
2) Freddo Frog chocolate caramel bars.

My sister Rachel had sent us pedometers, and for the first few days I monitored my usual routes just to see how many steps I was taking – it turned out to be around 6000 daily. Knowing that the goal is 10,000 steps per day, I've now made it my mission to reach that target every day.
If I have about 1000 steps to do, but nowhere to go, I march around the house with Ethan, we have a dance off, I run up and down the stairs as much as I can and generally keep moving until I hear the imaginary 'ding, sit down Mama'!
Then I reward myself with my beautiful small but chunky package of loveliness: Freddo Frog chocolate caramel bar. I really get a buzz from my little froggy friend and would gladly tackle anyone who tried to take him away from me! These have been my survival tools and I have inspired some of my non-RC friends to buy a pedometer of their own. Who needs a car when these legs can take me where I need to go?
The results are really taking shape now; I have lost a total of 20.75in, 2in off each thigh and 2in off each knee, 3.5in off my waist and 3in off my boobs.
I have lost a total of 17lb 14oz, and hubby has lost 20lb 14oz and he is so chuffed with himself!
We are now getting to a stage, where we will soon be lighter

than we have ever known each other and I am so excited about that. I pulled out my pre-pregnancy clothes from under the bed and everything fits me, it is such a fabulous feeling. That's after 17lb lost. What will I look like after another 17lb loss?

Blog 8

Today was weigh-in day for hubby and me and in my mind I had set myself up for a 2lb weight loss. I really wanted to get to 20lb off and even though my week had not been 100% perfect, I was confident I had done well.
So the moment of truth…I had lost 1lb 6oz…
In every respect, this was a great weight loss but my heart sank! I had so expected to see 2lb that nothing else mattered. I didn't congratulate myself on getting out of the 12 stones to the 11 stones or my inch loss. I focused on the numbers on the scales and felt rubbish. I'm 39 next week and I'd set myself a goal of losing 21lb before my birthday. I am so close, I can smell it and if I had lost that 2lb, I could relax a little this week and aim for the final 1lb.
I called my sister, as I do every Wednesday. We then played the 'how much did you lose?' game. From the tone of my voice, she assumed I had gained.
NO, I replied.
Stayed the same? NO.
1lb? NO
I've lost 1lb 6oz.
My sister was thrilled to bits and said 'What's the matter?' I explained my disappointment and she said something that really struck a chord with me! She told me I was doing brilliantly and that I was putting too much pressure on myself. It was great to have a goal but I should be proud of myself and if I tried too hard, I could jeopardise my weight

loss. Too much pressure can have a negative effect on the mind and cause you to eat the wrong things. My sister is so clever and so right! She also told me to exercise a little more and try to go for longer walks with Leo in the pram.

If I look back at my food diary, I can see where I could have done better.

So how have I done so far?

I have lost 1st 5lb 4oz in 51 days.
I have lost 24.4in all over.
My waist has gone from 35in to 32in.
My BMI has gone from 32 to 29.6.
My body fat has gone from 44.6% to 39.8%.
So, I do have a lot to be proud of and I promise I will not let the devil on my shoulder fill my head with self-doubt again. I *can* do this, it's not a race and I want results for life not just for this year.

Blog 9

FORGIVE ME, ROSEMARY, FOR I HAVE SINNED.
This is my first time in confession!
Last week from Monday until Thursday, I celebrated my 39th birthday with my lovely family and friends. This involved an overnight stay at a five-star hotel in London, a five-course meal and a very expensive bottle of wine, chocolate birthday cake, shared in bed with hubby at 10.30pm, a three-course meal in an Indian restaurant and a coffee morning at home with my amazing mummy friends.

In my defence I did, over that four-day period of celebration, make some very healthy choices but these were generally followed by some very unhealthy choices, ignoring the golden 5% fat or less rule. I'm not proud of my

actions and I am paying the price of my sinful ways. I feel bloated, lethargic and like I have let myself down. However, I did have an amazing time to remember and I feel my actions were fitting to celebrate my last year in my 30s. I hope you can find forgiveness for me, from within your enviable figure-hugging Lycra, and give me the strength to continue on my journey, undoing any harm I might have caused to my mission, this past blissful week!
Yours faithfully, Naomi

Yes, as much as I kid myself, I am not perfect! I really blew it last week and didn't even fill in my online diary for four days. At my coffee morning, there was so much cake, from carrot cake and treacle tart to fudge brownies and chocolate fudge cake…
I made it clear to my friends that no one was to leave until all the cakes were finished and whatever was left, was going home with them. They are the best friends ever, as everyone had on average four to six finger slices of various cakes. I literally force-fed my obliging 21 weeks' pregnant friend, although she didn't complain.
WHY, do we do it to ourselves?
I did my weigh-in as usual on Wednesday. I was pretty scared but I'm of the crowd of FACE THE FEAR AND DO IT ANYWAY. I was pleasantly surprised to find I had stayed the same. Huge sigh of relief. Put the weekly call through to my sister Rachel, with the results. She warned me to really be careful this next week as I could be in trouble. This was the day BEFORE cakegate. So as of Friday, I have been super-strict, hoping that by my next Wednesday weigh-in I might have un-done my naughty eating. I guess the moral of my tale this week is, to remember we are human and sometimes temptation gets in the way.

Blog 10

I have really abused my pedometer this past five days. The fab thing about my online service is I can see an average of everything. This includes average calories consumed, average fat, sugar and salt and average steps! I had been doing an average of 4000 steps when I first got my pedometer, and it really is a great tool to spur me on. My ultimate goal is 10,000 a day but I don't always achieve that. My average has gone up to 8000 though, so I am really pleased with that.

This week my mummy friends told me I was definitely looking slimmer. I have been wearing some jeans that my fit sister gave me a while back. When she used to wear them, I'd look at her admiringly and wished I could look like her too. Now, these same jeans are baggy on me, yes me! I am so excited.

My last weight was 11st 13lb, the scales read 11st 11lb. Woohoo, yippy doo, I lost two whole lumpy lbs. I am so ecstatic and happy that I didn't give in after my period of divulging!

So, that's a total of 21lb.

Then I got out my third new best friend, who I have hardly mentioned. This friend has helped me so much and it's a fantastic tool, exclusive to Rosemary Conley.

It has taught me to NOT FOCUS on the scales but the whole picture.

This friend is my Magic Measure®!

I used my Magic Measure® at the beginning for all my starting measurements. I hope you don't mind sharing my latest results.

I have rounded up/down to the nearest whole number and added my thigh, arms and knee measurements together, otherwise we'd be here all day.

TOTAL LOSS IN 65 DAYS
Arms: 5in
Boobs: 5.5in
Waist: 4in
Hips: 4in
Widest part: 3.5in
Thighs: 5in
Knees: 6in

That is quite a few inches and I feel fabulous! I even bought a size-12 buttoned top the other day, which I had first dismissed thinking it would never fit. Will probably wear it inside out to flash the label! I might even start wearing my Magic Measure® as a trendy new belt.
Hubby Alex, who was scared of the scales, last week, stepped on… He'd lost 4.2lb!
Men, how do they do it? That brings him to almost 26lb and major inches lost. He is pleasantly surprised how easy the Rosemary Conley plan is to follow.

Blog 11

Three weeks have passed – and a few more lbs have gone – since I wrote my last blog. They had their usual highs and lows but this week I have had one particular low that I will share with you. I have been mourning the loss of a dear friend, this friend went everywhere with me, including the toilet and sometimes even my bed. We went on long walks together and played hide and seek together and now they are gone. My life feels empty and I feel I have lost my weight-loss friend! Before you start to feel really sorry for me, I have to tell you I am mourning the loss of my dear, dear pedometer! She met a sticky end this week. Her back broke and that was it, there was no more data, no more clicking every time we walked together.

May my Polly Pedometer RIP.

I have been without her for a few days now and I honestly feel lost. I have empty spaces in my 'Steps' daily box online and it doesn't feel as if I'm following the plan 100% without this data.

There is a happy ending to this tale of woe; it came to me tonight in a vision. My sister has amazing foresight and had sent me an 'extra, just in case' pedometer with my original ones for Alex and myself!

So, tomorrow, I will be back in full fighting fit force. This pedometer will be called Pedro Pedometer and he shall be thrust upon my hip, to walk proudly with me wherever we go. Joking aside, this has been another tough week. I have found myself wanting to nibble, nibble, nibble. Damn you, emotional eating devil! By the time weigh-in day arrived I'd lost 2lb, which means I only have 1lb 4oz to go to the big 2st. Alex has 1lb left to go.

Also, I have 13lb left to go until I reach my first target of 10st 7lb. When I reach it, I am going to review whether to aim for 10st but I think that would be my final goal. I have never been so close to a weight-loss goal, yet I seem to be struggling with my willpower. It seems the closer I get, the harder I make it for myself. Thank goodness for the Rosemary Conley magazine and online articles. They always make me feel better and my thoughts and feelings clearer. I really do love this plan.

Blog 12

A wonderful thing happened this past week. My youngest son turned nine months and learned to clap his hands. So, every day I get huge dribble, toothy grins and applause from him everywhere I go.

It made me reflect on the past nine months and what a roller-coaster ride it's been. Then I started to look at photos and do some number crunching. I had reached 15st 11lb on the day I gave birth to my son. When I started Rosemary's diet, I was 13st 4lb 4oz so I'd lost some weight naturally in the first six months.

When I added it all up, I worked out I had lost over 4st in the nine months since Leo was born. That is totally crazy. How did I ever move about or get anything done? I know I was exhausted all the time and my legs hurt.

As always, my weigh-in day came on Wednesday. I had 1lb 4oz to lose to reach my 2st goal and I was praying for a result.

I removed my pyjamas, ring, watch and emptied my bladder – it all makes a difference you know! Moment of truth…11st 5lb 2oz. EXACTLY the same as last week. How can it be? Oh, I remember, I did have a few 'extra' high-fat treats in the week, didn't drink enough water and was not taking care of myself.

After two little weight gains, Alex took his turn, also stripping down to his birthday suit! I am sure my children think we are crazy. He too had stayed the same! His little face was so disappointed. We both lost a little bit on the inch department and had a discussion on where we were going slightly wrong.

We were both naked in the kitchen, chatting about our previous mishaps the week before and checking each other out. Alex has developed a two-pack! We are waiting for the other four to arrive to complete his six-pack. Alex was admiring my newly regained curves and commenting on my overall inch loss. Before you wonder where this story is leading, we got dressed and had our healthy breakfasts. We do have young children in the house, you know!

Blog 13

This week has been ANOTHER roller-coaster ride of emotions but this time with a happy ending. I have at last seen the light, hallelujah and all that. After my stay the same result last week, I started to comfort-eat again, feeling like I was just stuck and never going to finish losing the weight I wanted to lose.

I still ate my Rosemary meals but found myself snacking more and more in between meals.

I felt out of control and yucky, so I turned to my online gang and for the first time entered the 'coffee shop chatroom'. I found some other dieters who, like me, had plateaued and were feeling unhappy and out of control. I got six responses to my post.

Reading what everyone had to say helped me and it was suggested I should contact the online weight-loss coach, Janice. So I emailed her and she called me, on a weekend, and we discussed my situation. After speaking with her, I felt 100% happier. Basically, she explained when you have lost a good chunk of weight, you do plateau. It's your body's way of getting used to your new size and your brain needs time to catch up with the rest of you. This sounded reasonable to me and made sense.

Janice talked me through some ideas and I felt so much better and refocused. She recommended I have water with every meal, if possible. Yes, that is possible, I thought.

She also told me to be aware of my low points of the day and to plan to eat my Power Snacks at those points so I didn't pick unhealthy choices.

So all in all, since Monday I have eaten my three meals a day, two Power Snacks, one high-fat treat, one low-fat dessert and about three to four pints of water a day (some of this was from decaf tea). I have also cut my tea down to three or four cups instead of eight and when I finish my water, I fill the glass straight back up.

I got on the scales this morning and discovered I'd lost 2lb 12oz. So, in total I have lost 30lb! I got my 2st certificate and a little video message from Rosemary. I also lost 4 more inches and my waist is finally 29.something! I am so happy and excited. Alex also lost his previously gained 1lb and is back on track. I still don't think he is eating enough and I think he has realised this for himself now.

I am now only 9lb away from my first goal.

Blog 14

The unthinkable has happened. After straight weeks of losses and two stay-the-sames, I GAINED 1lb 4oz! I was beside myself, completely devastated. I had tarnished my perfect track record.

With a heavy heart, I took out my Magic Measure® and started measuring away. But all was not lost. When I entered all my measurements online, I had still managed to lose 3in! I called my sister Rachel, she could tell by the tone of my voice that I had gained weight. I was expecting her to tell me off or tease me (I am her sister, after all). She did none of this, but asked me some questions and said that from now on I would have to be 100% good, that I was only cheating myself and that the weight gain could be due to fluid retention from either my monthly cycle or the intense heat. That sounds good to me.

Joking aside, I ultimately am responsible for feeding myself and I knew I could be better. This past two months I have also been monitoring my monthly cycle. I was always regular as clockwork on a 30-day cycle but since having Leo, it's a 37-day cycle. Around the 16th day of my cycle, I feel ravenous and bloated. I also feel quite low and moody.

This lasts for about five days and it did coincide with my weigh-in. I don't want to make excuses but I did feel heavier. The scales just confirmed it.

So from that day on, I moved on to my Personal FAB Plan where I get to choose all my own main meals, Power Snacks, low-fat treats and high-fat treats! Up until now, I had tended to eat my way through the day and then add the food into my diary after I had eaten it. My sugar and salt levels were really high each day, so this had to change. I started entering in my day's food the night before, and then once I'd eaten it I added the time I ate it. This is really working for me. I am also doing 30–45 minutes of Wii Fit every other day and making the most of the sun and walking more and more. It has all paid off. I have found that in my life of chaos, it's great to be in complete control of my food plan. I haven't strayed at all and I've stuck to my chosen food rigidly, every day. When I weighed myself this week, it was a different story.

I'd lost 2lb 4oz and I am now 8lb 4oz away from my first goal of 10st 7lb. Plus I am almost the same weight as my slinky sister! This has not happened since the last man walked on the moon (that's not strictly true, but it has been a long time).

I am the lightest I have been ever, since my 20s probably. It's so nice to walk down the high street and receive nice comments from people. My husband and friends are such a support to me.

My new favourite thing!

It's called the Facial Flex® from Rosemary Conley.

Every night and morning, I am flexing the muscles in my face for a count of 120. It really makes your muscles ache but I honestly feel it's lifting my sagging jawline. In the first trimester of my second pregnancy, I suffered with Bell's

Palsy for about four weeks and the right side of my face dropped. It did return, but it's not quite the same and the Facial Flex® has also helped even out my face.

If you fancy a big treat, for a job well done, I highly recommend one. WARNING: you don't look very sexy while you're using it!

Blog 15

It's a few weeks since I wrote my last blog. But I am now back and back on track. Let me tell you the reason why I disappeared.

Rachel and I have a little sister in Australia and a horrible tragedy occured on 30th May. She was 38 weeks' pregnant and had just been for a sizing scan, when she had a minor car accident. Her huge tummy took the full force of the steering wheel and, sadly, she did not receive the correct care and attention she should have had at the hospital where she'd be taken in Perth, Australia. This resulted in her placenta rupturing and her gorgeous son Alfie Victor Smith was stillborn weighing 7lb 9oz.

My two boys and myself flew the long journey to Perth, with three days' notice, and attended Alfie's funeral and tried to do our best to ease their pain and suffering. My sister has another son who's a few weeks younger than my eldest, so they amused each other.

It was not all sad. We had a lovely mini holiday to the coast. It's the winter over there, so we saw quite a bit of rain but also saw some amazing sun rises and rainbows.

My sister's husband rented bikes and we all went cycling along the coast, Ethan and Leo for the first time, and they absolutely loved it.

During all this time, my Rosemary plan went out the window. My brother in law's mum made us delicious home-cooked food, such as roast pork with all the trimmings and home-made puddings. It would have been rude to say no…

Plus, after not drinking any alcohol since forever, I sampled quite a few local wines and loved them. My sister has very good taste and knowledge.

The flights both ways were HARD work on my own. Thankfully, I had lots of help and support from the air stewards and other passengers. One gent kept bringing me chocolate bars, saying 'I think you need this!'

All the way home, my trousers (now size 12!) felt tighter and I felt so sluggish and lethargic. I literally ate four Toblerone bars on the last 13½ hours of the flight to relieve my stress of non-sleeping children. At one point I had both of them on my lap, simultaneously crying and Ethan almost vomiting!

It has been a tough few weeks in many ways but I was so happy to be there for Amy and her family. She kept teasing me, saying I would be moaning about her in my blog and all the food and drink she made me have. But she did not force-feed me, I fed myself. It was fun but I was so happy to get home and get my food back on track.

It was so weird to not record all the food I was eating in my diary or plan menus. When I got home on Tuesday 19th in the late afternoon, hubby Alex had arranged for my weekly shopping delivery at 6pm. It was full of salad, veggies and protein. NO CHOCOLATE, CAKES or WINE. Home sweet home.

Wednesday was weigh-in day and I was half-tempted not to weigh, fearing the worst.

I swallowed my pride and jumped on the scales. I had gained…1lb. 1lb! How was that even possible? I felt like I had gained 7lb! I'd also gained 1½in.

So this week, I have tried my hardest to get back on track, knowing that all those chocolate bars could catch up with me! I have done some yoga and dusted off my Rosemary DVD. I spent 30 minutes in my living room with her, getting hot and sweaty! Hence to say, I haven't been able to move quite the same for the last three days!

So, a week later and I have good news to tell.

I've lost 1lb 10oz! That now makes a total of 2st 5lb 14oz. I am only 6lb from goal and I know now it's going to probably be the hardest 6lb ever, but I am ready for the challenge.

Alex also lost 2lb 10oz, bringing him back to a total of 31lb lost and me 34lb. I have also lost 44in all over and when I held up my Magic Measure® today, it's actually quite a moving visual to see exactly how much that is.

I feel fabulous and don't look too bad at last!

Blog 16

I know I say it every week but, boy, the past two weeks have been crazy!

There was no blog last week, due to my baby sister getting married! I managed for the first time ever to surprise her by turning up with my boys.

Rachel's civil wedding was supposed to be low key and simple to make everything legal, so that they could have a combined wedding/honeymoon abroad next year. That is still happening, by the way.

On Facebook, there were mentions of bouquets and buttonholes and the censored hen night photos, which I was unable to go to, so on Monday I decided to rent a car and come home for the weekend.

This little trip home also meant a little shopping trip to buy a new dress for the said occasion. I can't smile enough thinking about those few stolen moments while the eldest son was at preschool and youngest son was happily snoozing in his pram!

I tried on about seven different outfits and everything fitted first time! I don't remember – ever – another time when that happened. Oh and I forgot to mention, I lost another 2lb on last week's weigh-in. That made 2st 7lb 8oz!

So, after a little fashion show in Dorothy Perkins' fitting room, I decided on a flowery colourful number. I am beginning to love the 'shopping' feeling.

I also got a new bra. Alas, I couldn't afford the matching knickers. So I was fitted and lifted ready for Rachel's special day!

When I arrived, after Rachel's loudest scream ever, she hurled a vomit of abuse at me about how much weight I had lost and how skinny I looked. Bless her, revenge is sweet, sister dear! Ah, I am not mean. My only goal all my life was to look as great as my little sis.

At last, I am there and, dare I say it, 1lb lighter. Sorry, sis! All weekend, I was surrounded by lovely comments and went home with my head twice the size.

Can you guess what's coming next…? I was so happy, my emotional eating head raised its ugly self and all the way home with the boys we munched on chocolate and crisps. It also didn't help being the time of the month when I am worse, anyway. I have been craving rubbish all week.

So weigh-in day this past Wednesday was awful. I felt I had gained 7lb, by rights I should have. I had gained 1lb and I can feel every ounce.

Leo is teething like crazy and I am sleep-deprived again and wanting to feed all day long. Damn you hormones. I have resisted most of the time but my online diary is looking a mess. I have incomplete days and step records. Basically,

I am feeling out of control. I have 4lb to go until I reach my goal and I seem to be doing every thing I can to jeopardise my efforts? We humans are a crazy bunch! Some people would be doing all they could now to reach target, not me though. I am stuffing my face and it's got to STOP NOW!

Blog 17

Well, it may not be sunny outside but it is certainly sunny in the Mayer Baker household. Today is my eldest son's last day of preschool and I am sad yet excited for his future. I have officially changed my first major document (driver's licence) to my married name. It's only taken five years, but hey ho. Now to change passport, banks, insurances, everything! The list is never-ending.

So it seems our household is going through some major changes. One of those changes is my wardrobe.

It is now getting highly embarrassing wearing jeans that look as if I'm wearing a full dirty nappy underneath. Everything is hanging from my bum and looks ridiculous.

On Alex's day off on Tuesday, we sauntered past the Next sale. I had done a pre-scan quickly the previous day before enticing him into my trap.

I headed straight for the 16s and was looking through them when suddenly it dawned on me… I am not a 16 any more! I hastily searched for the 12s, which are normally full of clothes, while the 14s and 16s are rather sparse.

Now I can fit into a 12, was there much choice? Was there hell? Nnnnnooooooooooo.

This was my moment to shine but I didn't have much choice. I picked up some purple boyfriend cut trousers, red linens and a lime green top to wear with my white linens that I already have. I also picked up an orange pencil type dress, which I love.

All the trousers were fabulous and I strutted my way around Next while Alex was trying to control a very tired and grumpy Leo baby. He gave his opinions and indicated that he wanted to get me home to have his wicked way with me. I loved the dress but realised it wasn't very practical for my daily mum's wardrobe. I would look fabulous in the park, if we maybe lived in Richmond but not necessarily for Fleet! The one thing I loved more than anything was having clothes fit me straight off the hanger and the fact I'm choosing clothes with COLOUR, no black in sight.

Now, if I could only get a decent bra to fit, I would be sorted. I forgot to mention, the linens (without elasticated waist) are a size 10! I am going to wear them inside out, so that everyone can see, for the first time ever, I am a 10. I know it really does not matter but it was such a milestone moment for me.

This week I have also been doing Rosemary's daily fitness challenges, which she posts on Twitter and Facebook nightly. I have to say, they are quite hard and certainly spice up the ad breaks on TV. I especially like the running up and down the stairs ones, my heart races like mad.

Another thing I have been doing this week is having a double portion of my breakfast choice. I find I am ravenous in the morning and if I have two portions of branflakes instead of one, it really fills me up and stops me wasting calories on rubbish. We always seem to leave home so late in the mornings that we power-walk everywhere and I am sure I burn off my extra breakfast just on the school run.

Wednesday weigh-in day was epic! Was not sure what to expect but had 4lb 8oz left to get my target of 10st 7lb. The anticipation built, I stripped off everything and stepped on… Look straight up, I thought, nice and tall, pretend I am a giraffe.

Then I looked down. 10st 9lb 2oz! I had lost another 2lb 6oz!

I only have 2lb 2oz left to go.

I am so close, I have never reached a weight-loss goal in my life. I now know I CAN DO IT. My BMI started at 32 and now it's 25.4. I will need to get to 10st 5lb to get to 24 BMI but I am going to complete my first target and revise my goal from there. I can't believe the impact my weight loss has already had on my health and I can definitely run with Ethan now. Once Leo starts regularly sleeping through, there will be no stopping me.

I might even discover I have hidden superhuman powers and save the world.

OK, I know I am getting a bit carried away now but I hope you can sense how great I feel.

You all can achieve this, with a little bit of effort and dedication. I am not perfect, as you know, but I have accepted myself now for who I am and I hope I have learned to manage 'myself' forever!

I am coming home next Wednesday for almost two weeks and really looking forward to meeting everyone!

Blog 18

So, this is my last blog – for now. It's not a sad blog, it's a blog filled with excitement, disbelief and hope for the future. My excitement is due to the fact that, after 26 short weeks, I have met my first target. I have lost nearly 3st and I feel EPIC. In my working life before kids, I worked hard and got results and was rewarded accordingly. Since becoming a mum, I get rewarded with seeing first smiles, words, steps, etc., but I don't actually achieve anything for myself. Don't get me wrong, I'm not complaining but since becoming a Rosemary Conley addict, oops I mean member, I have felt that old feeling of excitement and reward. I have met a personal goal for me but the rewards extend way further than that. I have more energy, I can chase my boys and I can try clothes on that fit first time! My husband does not recognise me and keeps telling me how sexy I look. It's a wonderful, wonderful feeling and I want it never to stop. My feet have actually shrunk by two sizes! What is that about? I am still coming to terms with my new shape and the few times I have been shopping, I always pick up clothes that are too big. Also after being measured, I was shocked to find my boobies had gone from a 40E to 32F! I might use my old bras to hang my pegs in on the washing line.

My disbelief comes from what happened to me last week. I am still pinching myself now, wondering if it was all a lovely dream.

I was invited to Quorn House along with my fabulous sister, Rachel, to receive a makeover. We were with around seven other ladies, also receiving makeovers.

We met Rosemary herself (my heart was in my mouth) and she took us shopping one by one in Marks and Spencer, to find 'the outfit'. I tried on a lovely top and trousers and some dresses. Every time I stepped out of the changing room, Rosemary and her team were on hand to give the scores on the doors for the said outfit. A very fitted purple and black dress and black patent shoes were chosen for myself. Actually, I am jumping ahead a little. On meeting Rosemary she asked my size, to which I replied, a 12. She looked at me and said, 'Oh no, you are a lovely pear-shaped 10!' Oh no no, I said. Anyway, all the outfits that were collected were a 10 and, guess what, they fitted me! Rosemary really knows what she is talking about.

Then it was on to hair and make-up. In my life before

children, I was in the hair and beauty industry and really took it for granted. Since 2007 I have struggled to find a hairdresser that I love, and make-up only comes out for special occasions.

This was a proper treat and I felt like a trillion dollars. No longer a desperate housewife!

The photoshoot itself was fun but I am so happy I wasn't 'born' to be a model. It's so unnatural posing and smiling on cue. During the shoot, Rosemary teased my hair, placed my limbs and even lent me her lovely bracelet. She was very hands-on and encouraging.

Can't wait to see the photos!

Hope for the future: looking forward to new clothes, active holidays instead of the couch-potato ones I'm used to, teaching my children healthy habits for life and maintaining my current shape.

If anyone was ever in any doubt about losing weight, I would say DO IT. The Rosemary Conley plan is so simple and user-friendly for the whole family. It does not leave you hungry, you can still eat all your favourite foods in moderation and can go out to eat, without undoing all your hard work! The only person that can hold you back is yourself. If I can do it with my hectic lifestyle, anyone can. I cannot tell you how amazing it feels to be in a healthy BMI range. You need to experience it.

That's it from me for now. On to maintenance and I feel this is where the real work begins. I know I can do it, though. I am stronger than I ever believed.

Naomi

Your personal calorie allowance (women)

Check against your current weight and age range to find the ideal daily calorie allowance that will give you a healthy rate of weight loss after you've completed the initial 28-day plan.

Women aged 18–29			Women aged 30–59			Women aged 60–74		
Body Weight		(BMR)	Body Weight		(BMR)	Body Weight		(BMR)
Stones	Kilos	Calories	Stones	Kilos	Calories	Stones	Kilos	Calories
7	45	1147	7	45	1108	7	45	1048
7.5	48	1194	7.5	48	1144	7.5	48	1073
8	51	1241	8	51	1178	8	51	1099
8.5	54	1288	8.5	54	1211	8.5	54	1125
9	57	1335	9	57	1220	9	57	1151
9.5	60.5	1382	9.5	60.5	1287	9.5	60.5	1176
10	64	1430	10	64	1373	10	64	1202
10.5	67	1477	10.5	67	1389	10.5	67	1228
11	70	1524	11	70	1414	11	70	1254
11.5	73	1571	11.5	73	1440	11.5	73	1279
12	76	1618	12	76	1466	12	76	1305
12.5	80	1665	12.5	80	1492	12.5	80	1331
13	83	1712	13	83	1518	13	83	1357
13.5	86	1760	13.5	86	1544	13.5	86	1382
14	89	1807	14	89	1570	14	89	1408
14.5	92	1854	14.5	92	1595	14.5	92	1434
15	95.5	1901	15	95.5	1621	15	95.5	1460
15.5	99	1948	15.5	99	1647	15.5	99	1485
16	102	1995	16	102	1673	16	102	1511
16.5	105	2043	16.5	105	1699	16.5	105	1537
17	108	2090	17	108	1725	17	108	1563
17.5	111	2137	17.5	111	1751	17.5	111	1588
18	115	2184	18	115	1776	18	115	1614
18.5	118	2231	18.5	118	1802	18.5	118	1640
19	121	2278	19	121	1828	19	121	1666
19.5	124	2325	19.5	124	1854	19.5	124	1691
20	127	2373	20	127	1880	20	127	1717

Your personal calorie allowance (men)

Check against your current weight and age range to find the ideal daily calorie allowance that will give you a healthy rate of weight loss after you've completed the initial 28-day plan.

Men aged 18–29			Men aged 30–59			Men aged 60–74		
Body Weight		*(BMR)*	*Body Weight*		*(BMR)*	*Body Weight*		*(BMR)*
Stones	*Kilos*	*Calories*	*Stones*	*Kilos*	*Calories*	*Stones*	*Kilos*	*Calories*
7	45	1363	7	45	1324	7	45	1232
7.5	48	1411	7.5	48	1347	7.5	48	1270
8	51	1459	8	51	1387	8	51	1307
8.5	54	1507	8.5	54	1425	8.5	54	1345
9	57	1555	9	57	1480	9	57	1383
9.5	60.5	1602	9.5	60.5	1527	9.5	60.5	1421
10	64	1650	10	64	1590	10	64	1459
10.5	67	1698	10.5	67	1640	10.5	67	1497
11	70	1746	11	70	1676	11	70	1535
11.5	73	1794	11.5	73	1713	11.5	73	1573
12	76	1842	12	76	1749	12	76	1611
12.5	80	1890	12.5	80	1786	12.5	80	1649
13	83	1938	13	83	1822	13	83	1687
13.5	86	1986	13.5	86	1859	13.5	86	1725
14	89	2034	14	89	1895	14	89	1763
14.5	92	2082	14.5	92	1932	14.5	92	1801
15	95.5	2129	15	95.5	1968	15	95.5	1839
15.5	99	2177	15.5	99	2005	15.5	99	1877
16	102	2225	16	102	2041	16	102	1915
16.5	105	2273	16.5	105	2078	16.5	105	1953
17	108	2321	17	108	2114	17	108	1991
17.5	111	2369	17.5	111	2151	17.5	111	2028
18	115	2417	18	115	2187	18	115	2066
18.5	118	2465	18.5	118	2224	18.5	118	2104
19	121	2513	19	121	2260	19	121	2142
19.5	124	2561	19.5	124	2297	19.5	124	2180
20	127	2609	20	127	2333	20	127	2218

Index of recipes

"Portion control is key to weight loss and my **Portion Pots**® make measuring everyday food simple!"

Rosemary Conley

Rosemary Conley's Portion Pots® come in four different pot sizes with an easy guide that makes it quick and simple to measure your portions.

Available to order at WWW.ROSEMARYCONLEY.COM or CALL 08700 507 727 for our customer sales team

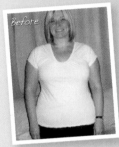
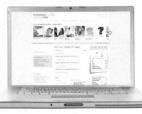

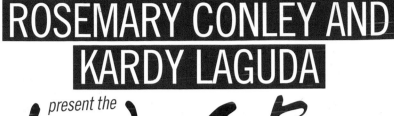
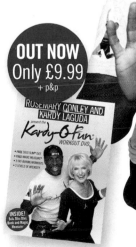

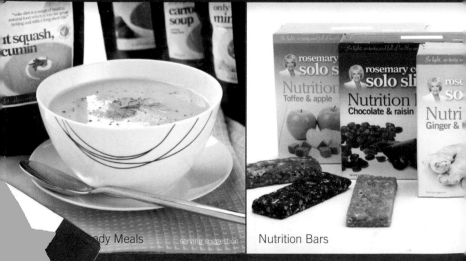